Six Steps to Effective Management series

Series editor: *Ann Young*

Managing the Business of Health Care
Edited by Julie Hyde and Frances Cooper

Managing Diversity and Inequality in Health Care
Edited by Carol Baxter

Managing and Implementing Decisions in Health Care
Edited by Ann Young and Mary Cooke

Managing Communication in Health Care
Edited by Mark Darley

Managing and Leading Innovation in Health Care
Edited by Elizabeth Howkins and Cynthia Thornton

Managing and Supporting People in Health Care
Edited by Julie Hyde and Michael J Cook

The *Six Steps to Effective Management* series comes at a time when the speed and extent of change within health care have rarely been greater, and the challenges facing nurses and everyone working within the health care sector are extensive. The series identifies and discusses those challenges and suggests ways of managing them. It aims to be unique in that it links theory with practice through the application of evidence where available and includes case studies which build on sound and relevant theoretical material.

All nurses are required by the clinical governance agenda to have a grasp of management principles. The *Six Steps to Effective Management* series is both practical enough to appeal to the practitioner and theoretical enough to be useful to those undertaking courses at undergraduate or diploma level. The books are relevant to all nurses.

The series comprises six volumes that are carefully constructed to contain a mix of theoretical and practical approaches, research and case studies, including a variety of perspectives from different sectors of health care. Each volume is relevant, realistic and practical to encourage reflection and critical thinking to prepare readers for flexible and adaptable styles of management.

Six Steps to **Effective Management**

Managing and Supporting People in Health Care

Commissioning Editor: Susan Young
Development Editor: Catherine Jackson
Project Controller: Jane Dingwall
Designer: Judith Wright

Six Steps to **Effective Management**

Managing and Supporting People in Health Care

Edited by

Julie Hyde
MA BA(Hons) RN RCNT RNT CertEd(FE) CertHSM FRSH MIHM MIMgt ILTM
Education, Policy and Management Consultant, UK

Michael J Cook
EdD MSc (Education Management) MSc (Quality Management) DipN (Lond)
CertEd RN RNT ILTM
Associate Dean, Learning and Teaching, St Bartholomew School of
Nursing and Midwifery, City University, London, UK

Foreword by

Margaret Goose
MA (Cantab) FHSM Hon MFPHM
Chief Executive, The Stroke Association, London

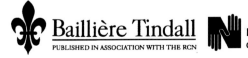

EDINBURGH LONDON NEW YORK OXFORD PHILADELPHIA ST LOUIS SYDNEY TORONTO 2004

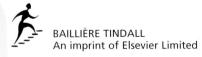

BAILLIÈRE TINDALL
An imprint of Elsevier Limited

First published 2004

ISBN 0 7020 2553 4

British Library Cataloguing in Publication Data
A catalogue record for this book is available from the British Library

Library of Congress Cataloging in Publication Data
A catalog record for this book is available from the Library of Congress

Notice
Medical knowledge is constantly changing. Standard safety precautions must be followed, but as new research and clinical experience broaden our knowledge, changes in treatment and drug therapy may become necessary or appropriate. Readers are advised to check the most current product information provided by the manufacturer of each drug to be administered to verify the recommended dose, the method and duration of administration, and contraindications. It is the responsibility of the practitioner, relying on experience and knowledge of the patient, to determine dosages and the best treatment for each individual patient. Neither the Publisher nor the editors assume any liability for any injury and/or damage to persons or property arising from this publication.

The Publisher

The publisher's policy is to use **paper manufactured from sustainable forests**

Printed in China by Elsevier

Contents

Six Steps to **Effective Management**

Contents

Contributors

Michael J Cook EdD MSc(Education Management) MSc(Quality Management) DipN (Lond) CertEd RN RNT ILTM
Associate Dean Learning and Teaching, St Bartholomew School of Nursing and Midwifery, City University, London, UK

Mary Gobbie PhD MA(Ed) DipN Ed DipN RGN
Head of Division of Critical Care Nursing, School of Nursing and Midwifery, University of Southampton, UK

Maggie Griffiths RGN BA(Hons) MsocSci
Portfolio Worker, UK

Barbara Hendry RGN DMS
People Development Consultant, UK

Alastair Hewison PhD MA BSc CertEd(FE) RN
Director of Postgraduate Studies, School of Health Sciences, The University of Birmingham

Julie Hyde MA BA(Hons) RN RCNT RNT CertEd(FE) Cert HSM FRSH MIHM MIMgt ILTM
Education, Policy and Management Consultant, UK

Nick Hyde BA(Hons)
Community Development Officer, Harlequins FC, London, UK

Debbie Lee RN DipN CIM MBA
Director, Developing You Ltd, UK

Jo Ouston
Principal, Jo Ouston & Co, London, UK

Application contributors

Julie Burgess RN DipN(London) MSc
Director of Nursing & Clinical Governance, North Bristol NHS Trust, Bristol, UK

Jeanette Clifton MA RN RHV
Health Visitor, Lewes, E. Sussex, UK

Sue Harris RN
Locality Development Manager, Birmingham and The Black Country Workforce Development Confederation, UK

Anna M Houston BSc(Hons) MA RN RM RHV
Research and Equality Development Officer, UK

Julie Hyde MA BA(Hons) RN RCNT RNT CertEd(FE) Cert HSM FRSH MIHM MIMgt ILTM
Education, Policy and Management Consultant, UK

Kate Jagger BEd PGDip(Management) RNT RCNT RN
Independent Consultant in Professional Development, KJC Consultancy, Kingston-upon-Hull, UK

Debra Larsen RGN ONC
Acute Pain Nurse, UK

Carol Marrow PhD MPhil BA DPSN CertEd, RMN RN
Senior Lecturer, St. Martin's College, Lancaster, UK

Christine Mullen RN BSc(Hons) MSc
Executive Director, Nursing & Quality, UK

E Nichols BSc RN RNMD CM
Head of Nursing, Medical Directorate, North Bristol NHS Trust, Bristol, UK

Tracy Packer RN
Nurse Consultant in Dementia Care (Acute Services), North Bristol NHS Trust, Bristol, UK

Mark Slattery RN
Senior Development Officer, Department of Health, Western Australia

Susan Smith MBA BSc(Hons) RN RM RHV Cert HE FWT
Programme Director, Centre for the Development of Nursing Policy and Practice, University of Leeds, UK

Foreword

Health care is predominantly a personal service given to individuals and their families, delivered within national and local health strategies. Thus the attitudes, behaviour, knowledge, skills and competency of the people delivering that care must be of a high standard if a quality service is to be achieved.

People working in health care do not come to work to tick off a list of tasks to be done. They come to work to feel that they contribute to making an individual, or group of individuals 'better' – either in the sense of curing illness through successful treatment, improving quality of life, preventing further ill health or by supporting relatives and friends of those who are ill.

This committed group of people deserves effective management, and the management of people is a key component of the manager's role. I welcome this important book in the series and cannot stress enough its importance from the patients' perspective – effective management equals effective health care.

The different sections of the book describe how to tackle this most challenging responsibility, and ask the readers to examine their knowledge and approach. Just as patients and carers are becoming better informed about health care and thus more questioning of our traditional methods of delivery, so too are staff becoming more informed and challenging about people management and the ways in which they wish to be treated by managers and to be involved in decision making about their work.

Management and leadership are different, but complementary. We should be encouraging the development of leaders throughout all staffing groups. Frequently I have seen an individual grow as a result of being given ownership of a project; it may be small in the overall picture, but he/she is able to make a significant improvement to an element of patient care. For example, the ward clerk who commented that there were too many forms and then set about amalgamating as many as possible. She designed new forms and persuaded her ward colleagues to use them, thus saving everyone's time and reducing the number of times the patient was asked the same details. This demonstrates real, pragmatic leadership ability that can really make a difference.

Foreword

Not all health care practice is about individuals giving care on a 'one to one' basis. Teamwork has always been key, but in many fields the development of more multidisciplinary and multi-agency teamwork is now an integral component of effective health care delivery. Indeed in the field in which I am now working – stroke care – the strongest evidence of effective stroke care is organised coordinated care delivered by a multidisciplinary team of stroke specialists.

Not all health care is delivered by paid staff. Increasingly the involvement of the voluntary sector means that managing people will also include volunteers; The Stroke Association has over 3000 volunteers enabling us to deliver Dysphasia and Family Support Services for our NHS and Social Services purchasers. Remember, they do not have to turn up each week, but they do in spite of the weather, family bereavements and other competing pressures. Why? Because of their personal commitment to the people they are helping. That motivation is widespread in health care and is much envied by colleagues in other work sectors. However, we cannot and should not trade on their goodwill.

It is satisfying to realise that the skills acquired in managing people in health care environments are transferable to any situation; health care workers are also members of family units, clubs and other groups. So, although this book is written in the context of health care, you can also read and use it to help with people management in other parts of your life. Similarly, when recruiting staff, don't forget that people who have taken a career break may have acquired good people management skills in the activities they have pursued.

Managing people can be demanding and frustrating but is, in my view, one of the most satisfying elements of a manager's role. It is only through developing others that good health care will be given. I have mentioned motivation and attitudes as key behaviours; please remember that this applies to managers also. Managers care about the patients, the service and their staff.

Margaret Goose
Chief Executive
The Stroke Association

2003

Preface

This book is the last in a series of six books addressing *Six Steps to Effective Management*. It focuses on the bedrock of management practice – *people*.

The pace of change is as fast now as ever it has been in health care, and the need for effective management and leadership has never been as great. Without effective management of people, service delivery cannot be optimised, nor can resources be realised effectively.

Whilst the fundamentals of people management remain the same, there has been a significant change in the context and scope of issues that impact upon the processes. Globalisation and the impact of world events on the economy influence management techniques and the workforce and its expectations.

Management is not a pure science – it is an eclectic combination of art, science, application and intuition. There are, however, some elements that are constant, even if their application has changed, and these elements are addressed in this book.

The book is divided into three sections, each addressing a broad theme. Section One focuses on the wider issues in management. Chapter One makes links with the impact of globalisation and the wider strategic agenda, whilst Chapter Two explores how working with a range of other professionals, often utilising new approach management styles, can add real value to the experience of the service user, and to those professionals delivering the service. This fresh approach is one that is encouraged by the latest Government directives within the influential Modernisation Agenda.

Section Two focuses on getting the job done – a crucial factor for all managers. Managers must always ensure that the job in hand is done efficiently, effectively, economically and safely to optimise resources and quality, and to minimise risk. Yet the only way to get the job done is to manage and support the prime resource – people – effectively. The three chapters focus on three important strands of management; managing change, managing performance, and the application of leadership and management techniques. These are pragmatic 'how to' chapters, and the applications take the chapter themes and tell real world examples of application.

Six Steps to **Effective Management**

Management is a complex and challenging activity, and thus managers, as any professionals, must invest time in themselves to ensure they are best prepared physically and psychologically to deal with whatever the job throws at them.

Section Three focuses on the elements of managing self in terms of self-maintenance and self-development. It is important that this is not done only via the route of formal courses that has developed, and gathered weight and popularity as we live in a credentialist society. The content of this section can be used by the managers to 'manage themselves' but also as a source of information and guidance when supporting the development of others.

As you read through the book, you may notice that some of the content of the chapters overlaps a little. This is deliberate, and makes the point that management and managing is not done in discrete parcels. There are enough theories of management, of change, of leadership to fill more than one library, so of course these cannot all be addressed in this book, nor is there just one approach to any one activity – for example that of change management. There are many variables and many contexts in which management of people is delivered – so the effective manager must have a shopping basket of skills and approaches to apply – managing and supporting people definitely is not a circumstance when 'one size fits all'.

We hope that you find this book a comfortable companion – one that you can refer to and dip into for a variety of reasons. We believe the content of it is real, and has pragmatic application in the fast changing world of health care. Supporting people and stewardship of the workforce is a challenge, yet a great privilege – good luck.

Julie Hyde
Michael J Cook

September 2003

MANAGING IN THE WIDER ENVIRONMENT – WORKING WITH OTHERS

OVERVIEW

The health care environment is a dynamic, fluid one, influenced by a number of factors. Three factors in particular must be considered:

1. Health care is not delivered in a vacuum so changes in society – and its expectations – must always be considered.

2. Health care is a political issue, whether or not that is considered by society as desirable. Elections are won or lost on the back of health care. Whilst governments come and go, those responsible for delivering and maintaining health care services must ensure continuity of service as the political tide ebbs and flows, and the politicians champion yet more initiatives and reporting systems to show their results for the next election.

OVERVIEW

3. Globalisation and the UK's links with mainland Europe emphasise that the world is a much smaller place. The effect of easier travel both in and out of the UK for staff and for the population in general, means that comparisons between health care systems are inevitable; such comparisons often act as a catalyst for change.

The dominant constant in this scenario is grounded in the workforce – the people that deliver the service. This means not only the clinical staff, but also the support staff, the managers, the volunteers and any group or individual who has a contribution to make to the health care environment. These people will come from a variety of cultures, backgrounds and experiences, and each will have a particular contribution to make. However, this will be enhanced and have greater impact if all pull together collectively to provide integrated, seamless care for the patients, clients and their friends and families. Thus if a manager is to be effective and efficient, it is important that the skills, knowledge and attitudes required to work respectfully with others are developmental and applied.

Managing in the wider environment

Chapter **One**

The influence of culture on the health care environment

Mary Gobbie

It is only through leadership that you can truly develop and nurture a culture that is adaptive to change (Kotter 1998, p. 166)

- Current challenges facing health care services
- Concept of culture in health care
- The healthy learning organisation/environment

- Emerging relationships
- Cultural leadership and management

OVERVIEW

In this opening chapter Gobbie identifies how effective managers and leaders influence the culture of the working environment. She identifies how the culture of a health care setting shapes the nature and quality of the patient experience, their visitors, staff and students. Gobbie presents useful theories within which to consider the organisation and delivery of care, staff motivation and lifelong learning. She shows how, by applying these theories effectively, one can use creativity and innovation to bring about positive changes to patient care.

INTRODUCTION

During the past few years the National Health Service (NHS) arguably has been involved in unparalleled change, flux and development. Organisationally, the NHS is trying to move from a traditional bureaucratic monopoly to a more responsive, flexible, needs-based and technological service. The original founding principles of free, equal and universal access to health care are now being challenged, reinterpreted or eroded (Green 2000, Social Affairs Unit 2000). For example there have been changes in the organisation and delivery of services (NHS Trusts, primary care trusts (PCTs) and the emergence of Workforce Confederations) and the financial charging mechanisms for dental services, prescriptions and personal care. Paradoxically, in the latter case political devolution has enabled Scotland to provide a more generous service provision for the elderly. Developments like this not only reflect altered perspectives on the nature and delivery of state-provided health services, but they are also shaped by, and shape, the established working practices and attitudes within the health services and the expectations and values of society. It is within this busy, challenging and fast moving environment that nurses are expected to develop and quality assure health care services through their leadership of staff and the effective management of the available resources. As Kotter (1998) argues, effective leadership acknowledges that in rapidly changing environments an organisation's ability to facilitate change is essential. This involves working with the various groups of people who comprise the organisation, understanding the external environment, the history and previous experiences of the NHS, and recognising the needs of the consumers.

The main focus of this chapter is to consider how the context and delivery of health care is influenced by what is known as the culture of the working environment. This involves an analysis of how the behaviours, values, beliefs and attitudes of the people who work in a health care setting contribute to a combined effect – known as the culture. It is the culture of a health care setting that not only shapes the nature and quality of the experience of the patient, visitor, employee or student, but can also significantly influence the working patterns, organisation and delivery of care, motivation, morale, learning, recovery and the ability to change, innovate and be creative. However, before considering culture, the chapter will first contextualise some of the current drivers for change in the health services. Understanding these factors enables nurses to be proactive rather than reactive in evolving more effective services. Following this review, we will

Managing in the wider environment

4

consider how the concepts of organisational culture, healthy, effective and learning organisations can be applied to the health care environment. Throughout the chapter, the contribution of the nurse leader/manager to the organisational culture will be discussed.

In summary this chapter will consider:

- the current challenges facing health care services
- the concept of culture as applied to health services
- what constitutes a healthy learning organisation/environment
- new and emergent relationships within the health services
- the role of leaders in 'cultural' leadership and management.

CURRENT CHALLENGES FACING HEALTH CARE SETTINGS

To identify the kinds of organisation that are best suited to the future health service, it is helpful to first contextualise some of the challenges and drivers that influence the structure of the current and future health services.

Current pressures for change come at three significant levels. First, there are the global/international drivers which may be economic (e.g. likelihood of war and its associations with recession); health related (e.g. World Health Organization targets, needs of migrants, changing epidemiology of diseases); and regulatory/legal factors (e.g. European Union working time directives, Human Rights Bill, freedom of movement). Second, changes at a national or regional level influence health care need and provision (e.g. devolution, policies originating from changes in government), plus epidemiology, demography and socioeconomic factors. Third, there are local demands which may arise from consumer pressure, local geography (urban versus rural) and cultural public health issues (e.g. incidence of teenage pregnancies). *The NHS Plan* (DoH 2000a) and the more detailed Wanless Report (2002) identify many of the global and international pressures which impact upon health care services and consequently upon the nursing and midwifery workforce (WHO 1995, Warr et al 1997, Warner et al 1998). For example, World Health Organization predictions and estimates to the year 2025 confirm the increasing rapidity of change and the uncertain and yet complex nature of health care development (WHO 1997). These developments include:

- reforms of the health services which include decentralisation, changing financing mechanisms, and greater participation of the private sector in the financing and provision of health care

- continuing problems with the numbers, deployment and working conditions of the nursing, health visiting and midwifery workforce
- an increased demand for nursing, health visiting and midwifery services, especially in community and public health settings
- the need for an increasing focus upon community care and research into rural and urban practice
- the importance of strengthening leadership at all levels in the health services.

Within the UK, the national plan for the NHS acknowledges the necessity for investment in staff and infrastructure with accompanying reform of the NHS (NHS Executive 2000). This modernising and reform agenda includes the development of new relationships, concordats, roles and responsibilities within and between governmental, independent and non-governmental agencies, professions, carers and health/social care settings (DoH 1999, NHS Executive 2000). A main plank of the government strategy is not only the demonstration of effective change through evaluated local action, but also its achievements through sound values (partnership, equity, fairness) and the dissemination of good practice. Meads & Ashcroft (2000) outlined what they consider to be a paradigm shift in the role of the health care professional. The health care professional is becoming more interprofessional (see Ch. 2), with clear responsibilities towards the design, planning organisation, delivery and evaluation of health care policy and practice.

Regulatory changes

Nursing, midwifery, health visiting and other health/social care professions are experiencing regulatory changes, which will impact upon the culture and practices of the delivery of care and the education and training of practitioners (DoH 2000a, 2000b). Current and future practitioners need to be appropriately skilled, adaptable, responsive and flexible if they are to effectively anticipate and respond to the new roles and competencies that will be expected of them. For example, consider how practitioners and students can best be prepared to:

- be board members of primary care trusts and other agencies
- be nurse/midwife consultants or other independent practitioners or fulfil the Chief Nursing Officer's ten key roles (DoH 1999, Wanless 2002)
- administer medications – by 2004 over 50% of nurses should be able to supply medicines (DoH 2000c, NHS Executive 2000)

● respond to the accelerating pace of scientific and technological change, the rapid obsolescence of knowledge and the accompanying ethical and professional challenges (e.g. gene therapy, cloning, multimedia, virtual learning organisations and NHS Direct)
● deliver high quality care at the least resource intensive level consistent with quality, the appropriate evidence base and undertaken by the correct competent person
● work in new ways not currently envisaged
● anticipate and respond to the cultural changes in society
● face the changing patterns of disease
● meet raised and altered public expectations
● meet new policy agendas – partnerships, quality issues, National Institute for Clinical Excellence (NICE), Cochrane, intermediate care, integrated services
● contribute to and evaluate evidence-based practice.

Workforce challenges

In addition to these drivers, nursing and midwifery face serious workforce challenges. Meadows et al (2000) in the introduction to their review of the NHS nursing shortage stated that 'the reason why a nurse may finally leave the NHS is often a "last straw", after years of frustrations and disempowerment, rather than a major cataclysmic event'. There is considerable evidence to demonstrate that the nature of the practice environment, quality of care, group cohesion and management style significantly influence recruitment, retention and ability to retrain staff (Levick & Jones 1996, Meadows et al 2000). The results of Levick & Jones, albeit an American study, identified the key factors related to management style were those which promoted participation, teamwork, mutual trust and confidence. Similar findings are evidenced in the work of Meadows et al (2000) who also noted that 'the history and continuing experience of organisational change was seen as unconducive to the factors supporting staff retention'.

Despite the increased demands for care and numerous recruitment campaigns, there are limited numbers of nurses available for employment. Two reasons for the static number of nurses available are:

1. an ageing nursing workforce with at least 10% of nurses being over 55 years, and 4.4% over 60
2. a reduction in the number of student nurses entering training during the 1990s (Seccombe & Smith 1997).

The Influence of culture on the health care environment

General patterns of employment include: shorter contracted hours in the private sector compared with the NHS; a gradual decline in the numbers working part-time (from 65% in 1992 to 59% in 1997); and approximately 25% of NHS nurses having a second job of which 11% is non-nursing work (Seccombe & Patch 1995, Seccombe & Smith 1997). Turnover rates are comparatively stable with approximately two-thirds of staff moving within the NHS system. These recruitment and retention factors influence the working environment and require innovative and visionary leadership.

As this brief summary demonstrates, leaders and managers within health service contexts are challenged not only by the necessity to change and evolve, but also by the management of the change itself so as to effectively support their staff. One way of doing this is to enable the staff 'to see their role as not just doing things the way they're designed today, but to figure out the way they ought to be done tomorrow' (Kotter 1998, p. 173). This means that leaders must understand the culture(s) of the organisations in which they work and thus enable their staff to participate appropriately in the evolution of different cultures.

CULTURES, ORGANISATIONS AND LEADERS

The concept of culture has its roots in anthropology where it refers to the customs and rituals that societies develop and exhibit. Unfortunately, as Ogbonna (1993) outlined, there is no consensus definition of culture! However, for the purpose of this chapter, it will be considered as 'the values, norms, beliefs and customs that an individual holds in common with members of a social unit or group' (Ogbonna 1993). You will see further reference to culture in Chapter Three. Since the 1970s, the concept has been applied to the way groups of people in an organisation act together. Groups have characteristics that are a feature of their members *as a whole*. This 'group effect' – known as the group culture – can be different from the actions of the individual members. For example, when patients refer to the atmosphere in a clinical area being 'friendly', 'peaceful', 'tense' or 'unhelpful', they are experiencing the cumulative effect of the staff behaviours and attitudes. Similarly, when trying to implement change that had been agreed by the staff as individuals (e.g. through a survey) a manager may be subsequently bewildered by the resistance to change which emerges from the staff as a group. As Yanow (2000) outlines, the concept of culture refers to both the characteristics of a group of people, and to the values, beliefs, attitudes,

Managing in the wider environment

meanings, acts (behaviours) and language they create together as a group. Some of these characteristics may be tacit or unconscious. For example, one clinical area may expect all the members of the shift to be ready for duty 5 minutes early while another one is characterised by a *laissez-faire* approach to timekeeping, starting and finishing shifts.

Schein (1992) describes organisational culture as the 'accumulated shared learning of a given group' which includes their behaviours, values, assumptions, attitudes and ways of thinking. In other words, the culture of a group reflects those things that the group members share in common and distinguishes them from other groups, or collections of people, who do not have the same shared experiences or values from which they can create 'culture'. When managing a new group, to understand the origins of their culture, the manager may need to ascertain some of their shared history and experiences to grasp why some of their behaviours, rituals and attitudes may have arisen. Typical factors to have influenced shared history might include ward mergers or closures, redundancies, relocations, a significant clinical incident with serious consequences, and behaviours of previous managers. Schein (1992) suggests that there are three levels in which the culture within an organisation may be embedded:

1. obvious behaviours and physical signs (e.g. the tenor of notices and instructions, general levels of courtesy, communication and standards of care)
2. a sense of what the group consider 'ought to be' their shared values
3. the 'taken for granted' assumptions about what is 'right'.

Inevitably, the third (deepest) level is hardest to ascertain and consequently change. As Ogbonna (1993) argues, the question is whether values and attitudes *can* be culturally managed and whether it is important to acknowledge that some consequences of cultural change may be uncontrollable and unpredicted. As Bennis (1998, p. 150) put it, to deal with the rapidity of change, future organisations will need to be 'unhinged': they will be 'confusing, chaotic places to work in' and 'full of surprises'.

Something is considered 'cultural' when a peer group applies pressure to an individual who has acted 'out of line' – perhaps being persistently late for work or continually advocating the overhaul of an established procedure. The group may apply sanctions – formally or informally – to the individual to indicate that they 'don't approve'. Culture includes what a group considers to be right, wrong, good or important; these characteristics are known as

The Influence of culture on the health care environment

the cultural norms for that group. The peer pressure to conform can be so strong that individuals may feel obliged to leave a group if they do not agree with the group's values and standards of practice. This is why people who become 'whistleblowers' may have faced victimisation if they have worked in a culture that refused to acknowledge or act upon reports of poor standards of behaviour or care. Where institutional racism or bullying exists it is often associated with particular cultural norms and tacit values and behaviours. In extreme cases these norms may lead to overt behaviours of discrimination and aggression (Meadows et al 2000). However, the tacit forms of discrimination are harder to identify and address. Wise managers will note patterns of wastage and recruitment in case they indicate inappropriate cultural influences at work (e.g. why is it that the bright/innovative/good/part-time ones seem to leave?).

Elements that may contribute to 'culture'

- Values, norms, beliefs, customs (standards of care, approaches to clients)
- Rituals (procedures and sequences of behaviour)
- Reward systems (formal and informal)
- Formal and informal communication structures (hierarchical, open networks)
- Daily practices (coffee before we start to check the patients or afterwards?)
- Organisational symbols (whether and what uniform to have).

Large organisations comprise many groups, and, as Bate (1994, cited in Hawkins 1997) questions, organisational culture should not be considered as a 'single unifying entity' because it involves complex social interactions. Morgan (1998) suggests that organisations are like mini-societies that have their own distinctive patterns of culture and subculture. Each subculture shows a pattern of beliefs and shared meaning, and exerts routine patterns of behaviours with norms and rituals. In the case of the NHS, several cultures, subcultures and tribes exist, be they nurses, midwives, surgeons, consultants, general practitioners, paramedics, porters or cleaners.

Health care settings can also influence the culture, environment and contexts of care. For example, contrast the working and care environments of an intensive care unit, an adolescent psychiatry unit, a labour ward and a residential home for elderly people with learning disabilities. Each of these settings differs in terms of length of client stay, the type and degree of dependency, the skill mix requirements, the resource allocation and the nature of care required.

Subcultures

Within a clinical environment, where staff are organised in nursing teams, there may be different subcultures between the teams. This is sometimes noted by variance in standards of care or 'atmosphere'. Patients, students and visitors often experience these differences.

Tribalism occurs when a group adopts defensive behaviours, often guarding information and controlling the work and relationships of the members and *excluding* others. Typically this is to protect the tribe's boundaries, market niche, income and working practices. Examples of this can be seen when nurses resist appropriate delegation to trained care workers or administrators or when medical staff refuse to allow nurses to instigate appropriate decision making in relation to client care. This attitude conflicts with the current goal that is about 'looking at the workforce in a different way, as teams of people rather than as different professional tribes' (DoH, 2000c, para 1.3, p. 9).

Interlocking cultures

Sometimes cultures may not always be 'distinct' because they may 'criss-cross' each other and interlock (Hawkins 1997). Cohesive interprofessional teams might be an example of this, when a new overarching culture emerges. Another feature of current workforce changes is new roles which cross boundaries, professionally, geographically and financially (nurse consultants, outreach teams, lecturer practitioners and specialist nurses who may work in primary, secondary and tertiary settings). These individuals can act as 'bridges' between the organisations in which they work, contributing cultural elements from one setting to another. Kotter (1998) argues that as organisations become increasingly 'boundaryless', it will be harder to develop culture and essential that effective leaders are sensitive to this and work to facilitate the development of the desired culture.

The seven S's

Organisational culture is of course not the only element that enables an organisation to be effective. Drawing on the work of

The Influence of culture on the health care environment

Six Steps to **Effective Management**

Waterman et al (1980), Iles (1997) proposes that organisational culture is one of seven interrelated companions of organisational effectiveness. Described as the seven S's, they are outlined in Box 1.1.

In other words, whether you are analysing the existing culture, or considering cultural change, it is important to identify and reflect upon those factors that interact with the culture. Strategies, for example, impact upon the way that services are delivered. These effects may be positive or negative. Meads & Ashcroft (2000, p. 37) compare strategies which can be associated with 'foresight, direction, purpose and success' and those which are 'flawed schemes, resource consuming exercises, unrealistic plans or a euphemism for exceedingly modest outcomes'. Whatever the strategy, there will be a potential impact upon the culture(s) within the organisation. Organisations that can sustain a positive and developmental environment are often referred to as 'healthy' and/or 'learning organisations'.

Box 1.1 The seven S's (adapted from Iles 1997)	
Factor	**Description**
Strategy	These are the activities that an organisation/group plans in order to anticipate or respond to changes external to the organisation, to the needs of the consumer and in relation to any competitors
Structure	These are the internal processes and mechanisms that enable the organisation to work. They comprise the allocation of tasks, their accountability trails, coordination and integration. An example would be the administrative, personnel and managerial divisions of the organisation
Systems	These are all the procedures and policies which enable the service to be delivered (e.g. finance, clinical, legal)
Style	This refers to the styles and values exhibited by the senior staff in relation to their leadership and management (e.g. democratic, punitive, hierarchical, *laissez-faire*)
Staff	This includes the numbers, deployment, competence and motivation of the staff
Skills	This refers to skills required to deliver the service and strategy (clinical/technical, interpersonal, managerial, research and reflection)
Shared values and beliefs	The culture of the organisation/group

HEALTHY LEARNING ORGANISATIONS, RELATIONSHIPS, LEADERSHIP AND CULTURE

From our previous discussions, we can see that the most effective, and therefore healthy, organisations are those that:

- can sustain a dynamic environment
- develop an empowered culture
- adapt and change to meet new demands
- have a strategic view
- energise people
- create organisational structures which allow the core activity of the group to be undertaken (Broome 1998).

These organisations are outward rather than inward looking, and focus on the customer (client and their carers) rather than the employee (Bennis 1998). Healthy cultures value initiative and leadership at all levels within the organisation (Kotter 1998). Kotter (1998) argues that it will be harder to develop cultures than in the past due to the changing boundaries, increased networks and the differing and changing distributions of staff. This is particularly relevant to the health service that comprises very large organisations. Meads & Ashcroft (2000, p. 62) suggest that (the then) level 1 and 2 primary care groups were to some extent 'virtual organisations' where participants had a sense of belonging away from the main employer or work site. This is likely to be true also in primary care trusts. As Kotter (1998) suggests, in these situations, multiple leaders are required to ensure that satellite areas can be led by people who are sensitive to culture.

Bennis (1998) outlines what he considers to be the role of leaders in achieving the cultural changes that are necessary. He proposes that effective leaders require particular attributes, namely they are people who:

- have a strongly defined sense of purpose
- have the capacity to create a meaningful vision which can be shared and articulated
- can live the vision (walk the talk)
- can generate trust
- can take risks, and try to learn from the experience
- can encourage bright people to work together and use their creativity
- can recreate their cultures
- can embrace change

● create the environment in which other people can be empowered to lead and take decisions.

For those who hold senior positions, this means being a 'leader among leaders' rather than a 'general' with 'troops' (Bennis 1998). This implies developing a culture with different types of relationship at a time when the NHS is experiencing a 'massive multiplication' in its relationships as a result of the new agenda (Meads & Ashcroft 2000).

Relational profiling, relational proximity

One way in which differences in culture are manifest is the manner in which the individuals and the groups comprising the culture interact and communicate. A useful tool to analyse this is *relational profiling* initially developed by Schluter & Lee (1993) and more recently applied to health service contexts by Meads et al (1999). Relational profiling works on the premise that relationships contain two aspects, namely *quality* (which refers to the how 'good or bad' the relationship is perceived to be by the people involved) and *structure* or *relational proximity* (which refers to the extent to which the persons know one another) (Schluter & Lee 1993).

While the quality of any relationship is essentially immeasurable, relational proximity may be quantified in terms of five indicators that are preconditions for positive, close relationships (Box 1.2). Relational approaches to health care advocate that the nature and quality of the relationships within and between organisations and individuals involved have a critical impact on their success and consequently upon public health.

Box 1.2 Applying the dimensions of relational proximity to health care cultures (adapted from Schluter & Lee 1993, Relationships Foundation 1996)

Indicator	Features
Directness	*The amount and type of communication*

● What is the usual medium of communication within and between groups? (e.g. memo, face to face, telephone)

● How effective is the channel of communication? (the accessibility and responsiveness of the groups to one another)

● How open is the communication? (the degree of clarity or distortion due to poor training or hidden agendas)

Box 1.2 – *continued*

Indicator	Features
Continuity	*The duration and regularity of contact*

Continuity
The duration and regularity of contact
- The amount, regularity and frequency of contact (shifts only meeting at handover, community teams only making contact by phone)
- The length of the relationship over time (whether those present now will be present for the implementation of change: the planning horizon)
- The stability of the relationship (staff turnover)

Multiplexity
Understanding the various contexts through which interaction occurs
- The extent of varied contact (e.g. the different contexts in which people meet: clinical, administrative, social)
- The knowledge and experience of each other and their work
- The extent to which the parties exchange information with one another

Parity
The level of mutual respect
- The degree of participation in the relationship (e.g. who is consulted before decisions are made?)
- The equality of the benefits in the relationship (rewards to all)
- Fairness in the way the relationship works (whether it is one sided, who exerts power, has and uses status or withholds information)

Commonality
The extent to which there is common purpose
- Whether the partners share common objectives
- Whether there is common understanding, values and beliefs from which decisions are made (shared culture or not)
- Whether there are common or different identities (tribalism)

The Influence of culture on the health care environment

Analysing the indicators identified in the relational profile enables managers to focus not only upon strengthening the relationships within and external to the organisation, but also provides them with potential strategies to influence the culture (e.g. relationships within and between staff and patients) and learn new habits.

The learning organisation

As we have seen, a healthy organisation is one that has the capacity to learn continually: a learning organisation. A model relevant to the NHS is that of Pedler et al (1997, p. 3) who defined the learning company as 'an organisation that facilitates the learning of all its members and *consciously* transforms itself *and its contexts'*. For Pedler et al (1997), 'company' refers to people engaged in a joint enterprise who 'accompany' one another and do things 'in company' in a collective endeavour. This requires structures and processes to facilitate not only the learning of the staff members as individuals, but more crucially the acknowledgement that 'individual learning is not the same as organisational learning' (p. xiv).

Yanow (2000) discusses how practitioners (in her case flute-makers) hold knowledge together and learn collectively through the activities in which they engage. In other words:

● clinical leaders and managers should analyse how the organisation *as a whole* can learn together so as to achieve the goals of the national organisation (e.g. NHS, BUPA), the goals of the local organisation(s) in which one is situated (e.g. primary care trust, general hospital, independent hospital, strategic health authority, home care team, residential home) and the goals of a small team of practitioners

● since nurses, midwives and health visitors work in the company of other professionals, managers and carers in a collective endeavour to accompany an individual through their experience of health and illness, this implies that not only do health care practitioners need to 'learn together for health' (WHO 1988, DoH 2001), but also that they should learn to work together

● in order to nurture and develop a specific working environment to evolve and become an integral part of the 'learning company', managers must be familiar with the structures and processes of organisational development, organisational culture and strategies to enable individuals and groups to relate effectively to one another.

Pedler et al (1997) consider that there are three evolutionary stages of the learning organisation: surviving, adapting and sustaining. Within each stage there are particular features which are summarised in Box 1.3. In the first stage, the organisation learns and exhibits behaviours which are focused upon survival, 'fire fighting' and acting habitually. From the survival stage, the organisation learns to adapt through its ability to accurately read and predict

Box 1.3 Key features associated with the various stages of the learning company (adapted from Pedler et al 1997)	

Stage of evolution	Features
1. Surviving	Offers stability, preserves learning and wisdom and useful procedures
	Firefights, operates in the here and now
	Employs habitual and automatic behaviours
	Can be rigid and thus finds innovation difficult
2. Adapting	Accurately reads current and future trends both internal and external to the organisation
	Adapts habits and culture to respond to trends
3. Sustaining	Achieves sustainable relationships with their environment and key stakeholders
	Contributes to the wider society through their positive relationships and partnerships with external agencies
	Has the ability to create their contexts as well as being shaped by them
	Incorporates elements of stages 1 and 2
	Can be conservative and adopt a 'survival at any cost' mentality with negative effects

internal and external developments, thereby effecting change to adjust to altered circumstances. In the third stage, the organisation creates its own contexts through sustainable development and nurturing effective mutual relationships with key external agencies. Where stage 3 is effective, the organisation operates simultaneously as a stage 1, 2 and 3 organisation, having the ability to contribute to the learning of the wider community, not just its own sphere.

As Pedler et al argue, stage 3 organisational learning incorporates individual, organisational and contextual learning. In the context of contemporary health care, a stage 3 organisation would be the one most able to adapt to changing contexts (political initiatives, PCTs, partnership councils), maintain meaningful work and development for its employees (good retention rates, healthy working environment and a positive skill mix) and develop sustainable relationships with other organisations so as to make a positive contribution to the wider society (social services, independent sector, non-governmental organisations, schools and workplaces). If the public health agenda is to be realised it could be argued that the organisation needs to be operating as an effective stage 3 learning company.

To consider how a manager can enable an organisation/working environment to evolve from stage 1 to stage 3, it is timely to consider *how* to change the culture.

STRATEGIES TO CHANGE THE CULTURE

Schein (1992) argues that organisational cultures are to some extent created by leaders who have to manage them, sometimes destroy them and, as Bennis (1998) would propose, recreate them. While not everyone agrees that cultures can change because they are underpinned by core values and beliefs, there are some models which assume that culture can be changed and managed. One such model is that of Silverzweig & Allen (1976) (in Ogbonna 1993). Box 1.4 adapts this four step model which has several key features. First, it assumes that when people come into regular and sustained interaction they hold a set of norms and expectations that influence the way the members act. Second, the group members not only shape the culture but are also capable of changing the culture of which they are a part. In step 3 the role of the leaders and managers is crucial in relation to their impact, role modelling, motivation and commitment to the desired change. This is why it is sometimes necessary to bring in a new leader with the skills necessary to lead and manage the desired change. Sometimes existing leaders are no longer able to manage the culture, the culture manages them!

At an early stage in the process, it is particularly helpful to consider those structures which may limit development, innovation and performance (e.g. adequate numbers of staff, working conditions, the scope to practise quality care, particular styles of leadership, the value given to education and training). It is likely that some degree of conflict or resistance to change may occur. This is to be expected, but one may not always be sure when and how it will appear. Open and trusting relationships are central to eliciting such resistance and identifying the overt and hidden agendas which need to be managed.

Managing in the wider environment

Box 1.4 Four steps to achieving cultural change (adapted from Silverzweig & Allen 1976 (in Ogbonna 1993), Iles 1997)

Step 1   *Analyse the culture*
- Identify the key features of the existing culture (e.g. survey existing members, involve stakeholders, ascertain the cultural elements mentioned in Box 1.1)
- Clarify and articulate the desired culture
- Identify the 'gap' between the existing norms and the desired norms
- Set objectives to achieve the desired culture
- Ascertain the strategies to enable the group to develop

Step 2   *Experience the desired culture*
- Involve all working teams
- Provide opportunities for group members to participate in establishing the desired culture
- Consider strategies to involve participants in relation to individual development, leadership, work groups

Step 3   *Modify the existing culture*
- Key emphasis on critical factors and effective leadership with good role modelling of desired behaviours (practise what you preach) and support of team leaders
- Work to influence the subcultures
- Modify the organisational structures to enable change (e.g. supervision, training, rewards, communication strategies, focus on goals, budget implications, policies and procedures)
- Instigate a systematic approach to behaviour change

Step 4   *Sustain the desired culture*
- Develop ongoing evaluation and feedback mechanisms
- If desired culture not achieved, review change programme

The Influence of culture on the health care environment

CONCLUSION

As Schein (1984, p. 15) aptly remarks, 'culture and leadership are two sides of the same coin'. In this chapter it has been clearly demonstrated that the 21st century requires new forms of service which in turn demand new organisational structures and cultures. This chapter has identified the characteristics of healthy working environments, which enable staff to learn, evolve and function effectively. These new types of culture and organisation need effective leaders at all levels. From Bennis (1998) it is recognised that what is needed are leaders who no longer operate with the old mindset of 'control, order and predict'. Rather, our future leaders will actually welcome change and see it as an opportunity, not a threat, confident that they can help to create the environments in which change and development can readily take place.

Practice checklist

- Keeping abreast with current and future drivers for change enables leaders and managers to anticipate and design relevant strategies for health care delivery.
- Understanding the groups and subcultures which comprise the organisation enables the leader to be culturally sensitive.
- Analysing culture identifies potential barriers and resources to effect change.
- Considering the seven S's alerts the leader to other factors which interrelate with the culture of the organisation.
- Cultural effects influence standards of care, recruitment and retention of staff and the way people relate to one another.
- Models of organisational development, cultural change and relational analysis can provide useful frameworks from which to lead and manage culture.
- Self and peer reflection upon the positive attributes of future leaders provides a platform for personal and professional development.

Managing in the wider environment

Discussion questions

- How realistic is it to ascertain the 'embedded values' within one of your groups?
- Consider how a manager could notice early signs of unacceptable cultural norms in a clinical area.
- Are there any 'untouchable' areas of culture in your organisation? If so, why do you think this is?

References

Bennis W 1998 Becoming a leader of leaders. In: Gibson R (ed.) Rethinking the future: rethinking business, principles, competition, control, leadership, markets and the world (revised edition). Nicolas Brealey, London, p 149–163

Broome A 1998 Managing change, 2nd edn. Macmillan, Basingstoke

Cochrane D, Conroy M, Crilly T, Rogers J 1999 The future health care workforce. The second report. University of Bournemouth, Bournemouth

Department of Health 1999 Making a difference: strengthening the nursing, midwifery and health visiting contribution to health and health care. Department of Health, London

Department of Health 2000a The NHS plan: a plan for investment, a plan for reform. Department of Health, London

Department of Health 2000b Meeting the challenge: the strategy for the allied health professions. Department of Health, London

Department of Health 2000c A health service of all the talents: report on the review of workforce planning. Department of Health, London

Department of Health 2001 Working together – learning together: a framework for lifelong learning in the NHS. Department of Health, London

Green D G 2000 Stakeholder health insurance. The Institute for the Study of Civic Society, London

Hawkins P 1997 Organisational culture: sailing between evangelism and complexity. Human Relations 50(4): 417–440

Iles V 1997 Really managing healthcare. Open University Press, Buckingham

Kotter J 1998 Cultures and coalitions. In: Gibson R (ed.) Rethinking the future: rethinking business, principles, competition, control, leadership, markets and the world (revised edition). Nicolas Brealey, London, p 164–178

Levick M L, Jones C B 1996 The nursing practice environment, staff retention and quality of care. Research in Nursing and Health 19: 331–343

Meadows S, Levenson R, Baeza J 2000 The last straw: explaining the NHS nursing shortage. King's Fund, London

Meads G, Ashcroft J 2000 Relationships in the NHS: bridging the gap. The Royal Society of Medicine Press, London

Meads G, Killoran A, Aschcroft J, Cornish Y 1999 Mixing oil and water. HEA Publications, London

The Influence of culture on the health care environment

Six Steps to **Effective Management**

Morgan G 1998 Images of organization, 2nd edn. Sage, London

NHS Executive 2000 Modernising regulations – the new Health Professions Council: a consultation document. NHS Executive, London

Ogbonna E 1993 Managing organisational culture: fantasy or reality? Human Resource Management Journal 3(2): 42–52

Pedler M, Burgoyne J, Boydell T 1997 The learning company: a strategy for sustainable development, 2nd edn. McGraw Hill, New York

Relationships Foundation 1996 Relational health care. Jubilee Centre, Cambridge

Schein E H 1984 Coming to a new awareness of organizational culture. Sloan Management Review 25(2): 3–16

Schein E H 1992 Organizational culture and leadership, 2nd edn. Josey-Bass, San Francisco

Schluter R, Lee D 1993 The R factor. Hodder and Stoughton, London

Seccombe I, Patch A 1995 Recruiting, retaining and rewarding qualified nurses in 1995. Institute for Employment Studies, University of Sussex, Brighton

Seccombe I, Smith G 1997 Taking part: registered nurses and the labour market. Institute for Employment Studies, University of Sussex, Brighton

Social Affairs Unit 2000 Overspending in the NHS: an analysis by 5 doctors. The Social Affairs Unit, London

Wanless D 2002 Securing our future health: taking a long term view. Final report. HM Treasury, London

Warner M, Longley M, Gould E, Picek A 1998 Health care futures 2010. Welsh Institute for Health and Social Care, University of Glamorgan, Pontypridd

Warr J, Gobbi M, Johnson S 1997 Expanding the nursing profession. Nursing Standard 12(31): 44–47

Waterman R H Jr, Peters T J, Philips J R 1980 Structure is not organisation. Business Horizons, June; Foundation for the School of Business, Indiana University

World Health Organization 1988 Learning together to work together for health. WHO, Geneva

World Health Organization 1995 Global advisory meeting on nursing and midwifery. WHO, Geneva

World Health Organization 1997 Global health situation analysis and predictions, 1950–2025 (Health Futures, 2025). WHO, Geneva

Yanow D 2000 Seeing organisational learning: a 'cultural' view. Organization 7(2): 247–268

Further reading

Broome A 1998 Managing change, 2nd edn. Macmillan, Basingstoke

Meads G, Ashcroft J 2000 Relationships in the NHS: bridging the gap. The Royal Society of Medicine Press, London

Workforce and Development Leadership Working Group 2000 Workforce and development: embodying leadership in the NHS. NHS Executive, London

Managing in the wider environment

Application **1:1**

Sue Harris

Clinical leadership

In this application Harris provides personal insights from her role as a manager, demonstrating how she applied some of the principles of effective clinical leadership within her own care environment.

INTRODUCTION

This application discusses the need for clinical leadership and explores the experiences of a participant who has both undertaken a leadership course and is now implementing it across a geographical locality.

Effective management within the clinical setting is of paramount importance to ensure the care of patients always remains the main focus of the practitioner. The role of clinical leader should be seen as a positive one, where the leader is able to relay skills to followers to ensure the patient is the focus. As Binnie (1998) states:

> A ward leader needs to be aware of the enormous influence their practice can have and to use it consciously and deliberately to inspire and guide others.

She goes on to explain:

> Role modelling is most effective when role models can also talk about their practice, explaining the thinking behind their expert work.

Traditionally ward managers have been appointed on the basis of their clinical expertise rather than their managerial or leadership competence. Performance management within the clinical setting comprises mainly staff appraisal and clinical supervision. When performed appropriately both these methods can be effective; however, due to lack of resources and education, the implementation of these methods is usually ineffective. Hence, performance management tends to become crisis management in relation to identification of training needs.

As a senior nurse it became apparent that the key to effective performance management is communication and effective allocation of resources. Ward managers need training and supervision in identifying training needs of staff in order to ensure the needs of the organisation and the individuals are focused to reflect the needs of the patient and the changing NHS.

Staff at all levels need to feel valued and in return will be more responsive to the needs of the patient and the organisation, thereby ensuring the main focus of all initiatives is the patient. The Audit Commission (1992) found that clinical leaders who fully mobilised all resources within the clinical area were more effective than those who did not. Research also shows that 'good leaders tended to produce good care and poor leaders tended to produce poor care' (Cunningham & Whitby 1997, p. 14). As a participant in the early Royal College of Nursing (RCN) Project for Leadership I discovered that if the team is working cohesively then the quality of patient care improves. I have since had experience of commissioning a team leadership programme across nine Trusts within the Black Country in the West Midlands. I remain convinced that an approach to performance management, incorporating a leader who continually engages their team and their patient in care delivery, is the most effective, and produces care of the highest quality.

As a senior nurse I was a participant in the RCN Ward Nursing Leadership Programme. I found this experience invaluable in that it taught me to focus on the team and the patient. Through the techniques taught I was able to identify strategies to help the staff evaluate their own performance. The initiatives used were simple, yet powerful, techniques of:

- patient storytelling
- observation of care
- action learning
- 360 degree feedback.

I now firmly believe that the role of ward manager is to enable the team to identify strategies and to enable the team to effectively benchmark themselves. The focus of performance management should therefore be the ward manager acting as a positive role model.

The focus of this chapter is therefore the influence of the leader on the team in relation to performance management.

DEFINING THE LEADER

The nature of clinical leadership has changed dramatically over the last 20 years. The Briggs Report (DHSS 1972) urged health care to move away from the hierarchical traditional styles of leadership and to move towards the development of teamwork. Yet it is evident today that this is still a concept that is being explored and recommended (RCN 1994). To accept the concept that teamwork is the basis for the future organisation of work then we must recognise the impact this has on the team and also on the client/patient.

Managing in the wider environment

Clinical leadership requires the application of many diverse skills, ranging from team player to strategist. Clinical leaders have responsibilities – legally and ethically – to their patients and the organisation that employs them.

The nursing code of conduct (Nursing and Midwifery Council 2002) ensures the public is protected through regulation and monitoring of nursing practice. Although it is the responsibility of individual practitioners to be accountable for their own professional practice, it is the additional responsibility of the clinical leader to ensure staff are performance managed.

Traditionally practitioners have been promoted to clinical leadership posts on the basis that they had attained a high level of expert practice. Although this is of value to patient care by ensuring practice is of high quality, what it does not ensure is that practitioners with the appropriate leadership qualities are thus employed.

A clinical leader in today's climate is the 'linchpin' of the organisation and the multidisciplinary team. The role of the clinical leader is paramount to the way in which the team functions. 'Leaders make things happen; they support, they strengthen and inspire trust' (Garbett 1998). Northcott (1997) however, warns that: Leaders are redundant without followers to inspire and mobilise, so those who follow must not be left out of the equation. These are truly inspiring words, but the question now is: How, as clinical leaders, do we make this happen? Leading people is a difficult task for any health professional and the assumption must be that clinical leaders should have appropriate support.

In their research into clinical leadership, the Royal College of Nursing (1997) stated that there should be support for newly appointed clinical leaders to assist them to explore their leadership styles and qualities. I would argue that it is imperative that this work starts at team leader level, so that upon promotion to departmental level, clinical leaders will be fully equipped and have the resources and support systems to survive both personally and professionally.

DEVELOPING LEADERSHIP WITHIN THE TEAM

In 1994 the Royal College of Nursing commissioned a 3-year programme entitled 'The Ward Nursing Leadership Project'. The impetus for the programme came from a shared belief that patients and their families should be able to expect high standards of care delivered by kind, understanding and professional nurses at the bedside (RCN 1994). The programme explored whether improvements could be made to patient care when ward leaders and senior nurses are facilitated to take more of a leadership role in their clinical areas and to promote patient centred care. The project aimed to promote better practice and to encourage ward leaders to become more effective by developing their leadership qualities through work-based learning.

The main principles of programmes such as this are to:

- enable clinical leaders to identify the skills they need to make themselves more effective
- demonstrate how these skills can be transferred to colleagues and patients.

Making a Difference (DoH 1999a) identifies leadership as an important issue and encourages nurse managers to cultivate this within their organisations. The role of the nurse leader could be instrumental in achieving the quality agenda for the new NHS.

PROMOTING CONTINUOUS PROFESSIONAL DEVELOPMENT

The advent of clinical governance has highlighted the importance of continuous professional development and lifelong learning and urged and encouraged practitioners to obtain user feedback in order to achieve quality services. Work-based learning enables both these aims to be achieved.

In 1996 the United Kingdom Central Council for Nursing, Midwifery and Health Visiting (UKCC) introduced Post Registration Education and Practice (PREP) which requires all practitioners to provide evidence of their ongoing development. It is therefore important that clinical leaders and managers explore with staff all avenues for ensuring that staff have update opportunities and that they comply with the PREP requirements.

Staff development can take different forms, from structured formal training to more innovative shadowing techniques. My own previous experience has taught me that work-based learning is a valuable means of promoting learning and development in the workplace. This personal view has been reiterated in The Peach Report (DoH 1999b) which highlights the need for education to be a shared philosophy of 50% practice and 50% educational theory. It is therefore imperative that clinical leaders remain clinically based, that they have credible clinical skills and that they are seen to be 'expert' in their field. As Benton (1998) states:

> Leadership is certainly not something that one can do on one's own. Leadership is about the engagement of others.

MANAGING CHANGE

On a personal level one has to agree that change management is a necessary component of effective leadership. It is imperative that to effect any development or quality issue within the workplace then the basic principles of change management must be adhered to or explored fully.

The main barriers to implementing new initiatives within the clinical setting appear to be linked to poor communication skills and poor change management skills. In my experience when questioned most practitioners can quote change management theory. The issue appears to be the practice–theory gap.

THE BLACK COUNTRY EXPERIENCE

The Black Country Education and Training Consortium has supported the local roll out of a clinical team leadership programme based upon the RCN programme. The programme targets team leaders within non-medical health care professions. At the time of writing 43 participants were half-way through their 2-year programme. These participants were influencing their own performance and that of their team by using techniques such as 360 degree feedback, patient perceptions of care and observation of care.

This technique of influencing change at a clinical level is effective, as demonstrated by these two quotes from participants undertaking the programme:

- 'Better care of clients, more interaction and engagement.'
- 'There has been a "change of culture" within the department.'

CONCLUSION

The question that remains worthy of exploration is: What makes an effective clinical leader? Despite several years of work and continuing research in this area, we do not appear to be any nearer the answer.

McCloskey & Molen (1987) argue:

> Leadership is the process of influencing people to accomplish goals, whereas management is moving an organisation toward achievement of its goals.

Malby (1998) argues that:

> The leader of the future will be able to think beyond tradition, will be visionary and will be balanced and intelligent.

Clinical leaders have a responsibility to their patients and their team to aspire to this ideal and to develop staff to achieve this. It is therefore imperative that clinical leaders are equipped to utilise all available resources for the benefit of the patient and the team.

Clinical leadership

References

Audit Commission 1992 Making best use of ward nursing resources. HMSO, London

Benton D 1998 Workforce planning. Nursing Management 4(9): 12–13

Binnie A 1998 How to grow more leaders. Nursing Times 94(28): 24–26

Cunningham G, Whitby E 1997 Power redistribution. Health Management September: 14–15

Department of Health 1999a Making a difference: strengthening the nursing, midwifery and health visiting contribution to health and health care. The Stationery Office, London

Department of Health 1999b Fitness for practice. The Peach Report. Department of Health, London

Department of Health and Social Security 1972 The Briggs Report. Report of the Committee on Nursing. HMSO, London

Garbett R 1998 United States . . . Marie Manthey . . . how nurse leaders at a clinical level could take control in a rapidly changing world. Nursing Times 94(28): 28–29

Malby B 1996 King's Fund ignites the leading lights. Nursing Management 2(8): 11–13

McCloskey J C, Molen M T 1987 Leadership in nursing. In: Fitzpatrick J J, Taunton R E, Benoliel J Q (eds). Annual review of nursing research. Springer, New York

Northcott N 1997 Pulling power. Nursing Times 93(51): 61

Nursing and Midwifery Council 2002 Code of professional conduct. NMC, London

Royal College of Nursing 1994 Ward nursing leadership project. Unpublished Report. RCN, London

Royal College of Nursing 1997 Ward leadership project: a journey to patient-centred leadership. Executive Summary. RCN, London

United Kingdom Central Council 1996 Guidelines for professional practice. UKCC, London

Managing in the wider environment

The supportive and facilitative manager

In this application Smith draws on her significant involvement
with and development of the Leading Empowered Organisations
(LEO) programme to highlight the importance of participative
and supportive leadership styles. The aim is to demonstrate the
value of this approach to front line nurse managers as a means
of achieving high standards of care. The LEO programme is a 3-
day leadership development programme which has been
delivered to thousands of health care staff within the United
Kingdom. The main aim of the programme is to enable staff to
lead more effectively and thus to enhance care provision.

BACKGROUND

Handy (1993) argues that front line managers have, over the past
25 years, received recognition for their role in industry. It is timely for
nurses to be given the same recognition in health care and the
opportunity to participate in finance, personnel and quality issues to
influence the changes necessary to meet challenges set out in *The
NHS Plan* (DoH 2000).

The NHS Plan 2000 addresses the public's concerns about the NHS.
The public called for:

- better paid staff
- reduced waiting times
- new ways of working
- care centred on patients
- better facilities
- better local services
- better treatment of NHS staff and the continuation of a national
  service.

The return of the Matron through the Modern Matron initiative aims
to put authority onto the wards, focusing on getting the basics right
without the need to be involved in organisational bureaucracy. These
demands were from the public, and policy makers are responding
(DoH 2000). *The New NHS: Modern, Dependable* (DoH 1997) and the

supporting strategies in three publications – *Information for Health* (DoH 1998a), *A First Class Service* (DoH 1998b) and *Working Together* (DoH 1998c) – together with the strategy for nursing *Making a Difference* (DoH 1999) suggest there is a need for improved leadership and management, and a more supportive, participative approach by management to achieve the changes. There are new structures proposed which indicate a flatter and more collaborative approach to delivering health care in the 21st century. Clearly there is an expectation that by increasing the responsibilities of front line ward managers the problems of discharge delays and cleanliness of the environment will be solved.

STRUCTURES AND SYSTEMS NEED TO SUPPORT THE PARTICIPATION PROCESS

Rosabeth Moss Kanter (1990) suggests the complexity of change requires a move away from the archetypal image of leaders as heroes. She calls for organisations to reassess their corporate structures and put in place systems that create synergies, partnership and cooperation.

In American and UK health care organisations, the creation of synergies in nursing has been adopted by the introduction of shared governance (Porter-O'Grady 1992). This is a mechanism by which professional nurses work in collaboration to accomplish their clinical practice outcomes and influence finance, personnel and quality. Front line managers and nurses participate in all related activities that support nursing practice such as development of standards, quality improvements research, education and management (McDonagh et al 1989). Shared governance requires increased participation, at all levels of nursing, in the decision-making process through participation on councils and committees. A global perspective of the organisation is thus developed to enable problems and concerns to be collectively addressed.

USING THEORY TO IMPROVE MANAGEMENT AND LEADERSHIP

To enhance the ability of staff to manage and lead more effectively some knowledge of related theory is useful. McNichol (2000), however, suggests that a common weakness of theories is that much of their value is lost through a failure to translate the concepts into a practical model. The LEO programme provides a practical framework and draws examples from the participants that help demonstrate practical application of the theories to practise. Many authors suggest management and leadership should be seen as the same

Yukl (1994). Miller and Manthey (2000), developers of the LEO programme, disagree and argue there needs to be a distinction made between management and leadership. The distinction lies in the willingness of the manager to learn the art of effective leadership:

> Everyone in a managerial position is perforce a leader, this is not a choice. The choice is whether you are skilled or unskilled. (Manthey and Miller 2000 `Leading an Empowered Organisation' Training Manual.)

If the goal is to assist front line nurse managers in adopting an approach to management and leadership that will address the concerns of the public, then there will be new skills to learn. Handy (1995) argues that it is important to address the individual approach to management, particularly in the fast changing environment of the last decade. The management and leadership of groups is a vital ingredient in the effectiveness of organisation of other staff.

LEADERS AND FOLLOWERS IN A SELF-MANAGEMENT PROCESS

Kelly (1998) suggests that the effectiveness of the leader is determined by the interaction of the follower with the leader. The follower has a responsibility to contribute to the effectiveness of the leader. Followers need the following qualities:

- to manage themselves well
- to be committed to the organisation's purpose and principles
- to build their competence
- to be courageous, honest and credible.

The effective follower therefore engages in a process of self-management. The leader's function is to cultivate effective self-management. In groups of professional people the equality of leader and follower needs to be emphasised.

The distinguishing feature between leader and follower is the role each plays. The leader has vision and creates strategies to realise the vision, has effective interpersonal skills to achieve consensus, can communicate and enthuse groups, and is able to coordinate disparate efforts. The follower also needs vision and the social capacity to work with others, to pursue his/her own goals (but not at the cost of others) and to work within a common purpose.

Kelly (1998) reinforces the need for peer and boss feedback systems, suggesting all workers in organisations are leaders and followers, and that it is the role function that determines the emphasis placed on leadership of a group. Pittman et al (1998) argue that research in both public and private organisations strongly suggests that there are two fundamental dimensions of follower initiative: *performance initiative* (which refers to the follower's active attempt to be effective) and *relationship initiative* (which relates to the active attempt by the follower to work on the relationship). For effective partnership, there is a need for a high degree of both performance and relationship initiative.

To develop partnerships in organisations the following activities need to be in place:

- Skills development in communication and problem solving
- Support and rewards for people who develop relationship initiatives
- Selection systems that look for competence in relationship building and people who are willing to develop such skills.

ORGANISATIONS AS COMPLEX OPEN SYSTEMS

Systems theory provides a model to explore the behaviours of people within subsystems and the nature of the relationships across boundaries. It also provides a model of the technical and social aspects of the organisation and the individual within the group. Changing one component in an open system will have a knock-on effect in many others.

Theories of leadership and management developed over the last hundred years assume a stable environment and subsystems that do not change. The scientific rational models of leadership and management tend to focus on the technical and social subsystems of organisations without attention to conflicting subsystems (Lawrence & Lorsch 1967).

Stacey (2002) insists that the rational models of leadership and management fail to take account of the psychoanalytical processes that occur in groups. Individuals unaware of their own behaviour will impact on the culture. The management and leadership scenario does not take place in a vacuum – it is a dynamic and chaotic process. It is fragile and the reality of organisational life is that it is ambiguous and uncertain.

Stacey (2002) suggests too that all managers are participants in a dynamic process of interaction. Despite the desire to provide intentional direction through strategy and policy formulation, the process of participation results in unexpected responses.

Senge (1990) describes the need for new roles and skills for leaders and managers who need to deal with the chaos and complexity of change. The need for interdependence across boundaries requires all managers and leaders to be creators, teachers and stewards. These roles require new skills, such as the ability to:

- build a shared vision
- bring to the surface and challenge the prevailing mental models
- foster more systematic patterns of thinking.

Senge refers to the need for a 'learning organisation' where people expand their capabilities to shape the future and leaders become responsible for learning.

Organisational learning takes place through a process of interaction. Most organisations are made up of work groups. Some are referred to as teams, others as functional work units. NHS structures are diverse and complex, the unifying aspect being 'diversity'. As Handy (1995) points out, the success stories of yesterday have little relevance to the problems of tomorrow, they might even be damaging. The front line nurse leaders and managers of today must look forward not backward, think creatively and differently, take risks and make mistakes. The work place is a place of chaos, creativity and complexity, fired with excitement and fun.

Handy (1995) acknowledges that this way of thinking results in the need to give individuals more freedom, with which they may not be comfortable; most people are not comfortable or ready to tolerate this level of ambiguity. Translating the truisms into recipes for action for front line managers is not easy. In collaborative systems there is always the need for finding the balance between compromise, the corporate need for control and the individual need for autonomy. The LEO programme provides an environment where leaders can explore these boundaries and determine approaches that will work well in their environment.

References

Department of Health 1997 The new NHS: modern, dependable. Session 1997–98; Cm 3807. The Stationery Office, London

Department of Health 1998a Information for health: an information strategy for the modern NHS 1998–2005. NHS Executive, Leeds

Department of Health 1998b A first class service: quality in the new NHS. Department of Health, London

Department of Health 1998c The new NHS – working together: securing a quality workforce for the NHS. Department of Health, London

Department of Health 1999 Making a difference, strengthening the nursing, midwifery and health visiting contribution to health and healthcare. Department of Health, London

Department of Health 2000 The NHS plan – a plan for investment, a plan for reform. Department of Health, London

Handy C 1993 Understanding organisations, 4th edn. Penguin, London

Handy C 1995 Beyond certainty. Hutchinson, London

Kelly R 1998 In praise of followers. In: Rosenbach W E, Taylor R L (eds) Contemporary issues in leadership. West View Press, Boulder, Colorado

Lawrence P R, Lorsch J W 1967 Organisation and environment. Harvard University Press, Cambridge, MA

McDonagh K J, Rhodes B, Sharkey K, Goodroe J H 1989 Shared governance at St Joseph's Hospital of Atlanta: 'a mature professional practice model'. Nursing Administration Quarterly 13(4): 17–28

The supportive and facilitative manager

Six Steps to **Effective Management**

McNichol E 2000 How to be a model leader. Nursing Standard 14(45): 24

Manthey M, Miller D 2000 Leading an empowered organisation. Training Manual, Creative Healthcare Consultants, Minneapolis

Moss Kanter R 1990 When giants learn to dance. Simon and Schuster, New York

Pittman T S, Rosenbach W E, Potter E H 1998 Followers as partners. In: Rosenbach W E, Taylor R L (eds) Contemporary issues in leadership. West View Press, Boulder, Colorado

Porter-O'Grady T (ed.) 1992 Implementing shared governance, creating a professional organisation. Mosby Year Book, St Louis, MO

Senge P 1990 The fifth discipline: the art and practice of the learning organisation. Doubleday/Currency, New York

Stacey R D 2002 Strategic management and organisational dynamics, 4th edn. Prentice Hall, Harlow

Yukl G 1994 Leadership in organizations, 3rd edn. Prentice Hall International, Englewood Cliffs, NJ

Managing in the wider environment

Chapter **Two**

How to work with other professionals:

multiprofessional and collaborative working

Maggie Griffiths and Alistair Hewison

- What is a team?
- What is a multidisciplinary team?
- Theories of teamwork

- Multiprofessional working in health care
- The reality of achieving teamworking

OVERVIEW

In this chapter Griffiths and Hewison identify key issues relating to working between teams and across boundaries. They point out that within the literature authors do not use the terminology consistently. This is further complicated by the Department of Health's recent shift to using the term 'common learning'. Common learning in this context is being used to describe any activity that involves staff from several different groups working or learning together. Readers that require more detailed definitions and further reading are advised to consult the website at the Centre for the Advancement of Interprofessional Education (CAIPE) www.caipe.org.uk.

INTRODUCTION

The importance of teamworking has been emphasised in a series of policy documents as an essential feature of effective health care delivery (DoH 1996a, 1996b, 1996c). This has been taken forward in *The NHS Plan* (DoH 2000a) and in the paper reporting on progress made as a result of increasing the number of staff in the NHS (DoH 2001) which calls for more teamworking, extended roles for professionals and the removal of obstacles to collaboration. In a general sense, people talk about teamwork when they want to emphasise the virtues of cooperation and the need to make use of the strengths of employees (Mullins 2002) and although it has long been regarded as the best way of organising work in health care settings, it is only relatively recently that evidence has emerged to support this assumption. Carter & West (1999), for example, have found that teamworking reduces stress in team members and West, in a series of studies, has established that effective teamworking reduces patient mortality (Borrill et al 2001, West 2002). For these reasons alone it is important that nurses understand how and why teams work. This takes on added significance if it is considered that the *Improving Working Lives* initiative (DoH 2000b) and multiprofessional and collaborative working between a range of staff in health and social care, are also founded on teamwork.

However, getting people to work in teams can be difficult and there are many barriers to overcome. These include lack of agreement on common aims among team members, 'tribalism' and organisational factors (English National Board 1997). This is compounded by the fact that teams in health care vary considerably in terms of their size, composition and function; consequently there are no universal 'rules' that can be applied to bring about effective teamwork. Yet this does not make multiprofessional working impossible (Firth-Cozens 2001).

Outline

The purpose of this chapter is to examine the theory of teams and combine this with some practical examples in order to demonstrate the sort of things that need to be addressed when building multiprofessional teams. There is no 'quick fix'; teamworking of this nature requires careful application of theoretical principles whilst taking account of the specific local circumstances and requirements. The chapter is divided into sections, each of which addresses an important element of multiprofessional teamwork in

Managing in the wider environment

> **Box 2.1** Learning outcomes
>
> When you have read this chapter you should be able to:
> - define the term 'team'
> - summarise the theoretical basis of effective teamwork
> - compare and contrast the terms 'multiprofessional', 'interprofessional' and 'interdisciplinary'
> - apply theories of teamwork to the reality of practice in the NHS.

health care. First it is necessary to examine the terminology involved: teamwork, multidisciplinary teams, interprofessional working and interagency collaboration have all become part of language of the NHS, yet what do these terms mean? Next some of the main principles of effective teamworking that have emerged from the literature will be summarised and related to health care. This will be followed by a more detailed consideration of the work that has focused on multidisciplinary teamworking to ensure the specific issues related to health care are discussed. Finally comment will be made on the practicalities involved in building teams in a complex and changing environment. Learning outcomes from this chapter are summarised in Box 2.1.

WHAT IS TEAMWORK?

A team can be defined as:

> ... a group with a sense of common goal or task, the pursuit of which requires collaboration and the coordination of the activities of its members, who have regular and frequent interaction with one another. (Martin & Henderson 2001, p. 93)

Yet this only takes us so far. How does this apply to your work setting? It is likely that you are in more than one team and that you have different roles in the different teams in which you work. Do they operate in the same way?

Another issue to consider is the mix of professionals in the team. The collaboration that is required in contemporary health care involves contributions from a range of health care professionals, as well as managers and colleagues working in social services, local government and the voluntary sector. The organisations these team members work for often have different structures, reporting mechanisms and cultures, all of which have an effect on teamwork.

The size of the team is also important. The maximum team size for 'optimum' performance may be 12, yet in the NHS most teams exceed this number (Carter & West 1999). Health care teams are also often geographically dispersed and may have no common base building to meet in. Indeed some team members may meet so rarely that conventional notions of team meetings become impractical. This suggests that some other means of defining multiprofessional teamwork is needed. However this is by no means straightforward either. The precise meaning of the terms employed in this area is not clear. Prefixes such as inter-, multi- and trans- are used randomly and in different contexts and the descriptions in the professional literature are so diverse that their meaning is 'murky' (McCallin 2001).

The use of these terms has also been challenged on the basis that there is little evidence of the cost effectiveness of these approaches when compared with services delivered by the separate professions (Øvretveit 1997). Perhaps more importantly it has also been suggested that there is scant evidence to substantiate the view that collaboration leads to an increase in the quality of care which has furthered the wellbeing of patients (Leathard 1994). The work of West (2002), mentioned earlier, provides evidence which addresses these concerns. Despite this, however, the imprecise terminology persists. The terms continue to be used widely and regular calls for more multidisciplinary teamwork and interdisciplinary working are made. In view of this it is important to examine the definitions that have been developed so that those responsible for building and managing such teams are aware of what is involved.

Øvretveit suggests:

> A general definition of a multidisciplinary team is: a group of practitioners with different professional training (multidisciplinary), employed by more than one agency (multiagency), who meet regularly to coordinate their work providing services to one or more clients in a defined area. (Øvretveit 1993, p. 9)

whereas Leathard (1994) argues that interdisciplinary practice refers to people with distinct disciplinary training working together for a common purpose, as they make different yet complementary contributions to patient-focused care. These definitions are fairly similar although they are ostensibly referring to two different terms. In view of this lack of agreement surrounding the terms involved it is probably more beneficial to focus on the main issues associated with this area rather than seeking an elusive comprehensive definition. Some useful work that has examined this area is summarised below.

INTERPROFESSIONAL WORKING

It has been established that interprofessional and multiprofessional working are issues of concern and have been advocated as ways of organising work in health care. However, there is a need to look beyond the terms to understand what working in this way entails. Davis (1988) suggests that learning to work with others can be seen as taking place on a continuum of growth. This continuum is made up of the levels of interprofessional work outlined in Box 2.2.

Different groups of professionals and teams will be at different points on this continuum and this will affect the way they operate. Øvretveit (1997) suggests that a more fruitful approach in developing understanding of the nature of interprofessional working is to consider the different types of interprofessional working that exist and use this to design and improve interprofessional working arrangements. This is an important point as it underlines the observation made earlier that there is no set prescription for multiprofessional working. Different arrangements will need to be put in place in different settings if the team is to be successful. Essentially those working in and/or responsible for such teams can identify which type of team they are in or wish to build.

Multiprofessional working then is not a single entity. There will be different arrangements, team members, reporting mechanisms and criteria for success depending on the purpose of the team. For example, a multidisciplinary team on a ward in an acute trust is likely to include the nurse(s), a physiotherapist, an occupational therapist, a doctor, a dietitian, and a social worker, amongst others. Although each team member is working to care for the patients on

---

Box 2.2   Levels of interprofessional work

Unidisciplinarity Feeling confident and competent in one's own discipline.

Intradisciplinarity Believing that you and fellow professionals in your own discipline can make an important contribution to care.

Multidisciplinarity Recognising that other disciplines also have important contributions to make.

Interdisciplinarity Willing and able to work with others in the joint evaluation, planning and care of the patient.

Transdisciplinarity Making the commitment to teach and practice with other disciplines across traditional boundaries for the benefit of the patient's immediate needs.

How to work with other professionals

that particular ward, they are not all managed by the same person. Each individual is likely to have a different line manager. The professionals involved are also accountable to a professional head of their particular service. Consequently, even before the team sets out to do anything, there are factors present that can work against cohesiveness.

When thinking about teams in general there is an identified leader and the task is clear. However, in multidisciplinary teams the leadership can vary, depending on the task or issue, and there is a separate line of accountability to a professional head which exists alongside the managerial accountability of the team. If it is then considered that different team members may have different views of the task, arising from their professional background, it becomes clear why 'standard' prescriptions for teamwork need to be modified. There can be disagreements concerning what the team should focus on. It may be that a patient is deemed 'medically fit' and so should be discharged, whereas other members of the team may believe that more time is needed for recovery before discharge.

Similarly the working arrangements of the different professionals within the team can combine to prevent the provision of coordinated care. Physiotherapists and occupational therapists visiting the ward may have limited 'time slots' and come to work with patients who are still tired after having had a wash. The visit is scheduled at this time because the therapists have other commitments during the day. This disrupts the care planned by the nurse. These circumstances indicate that if multidisciplinary teamworking is to be achieved, time and effort need to be devoted to it.

If this is to happen and the decisions that Øvretveit (1997) refers to are to be made, it is helpful if team leaders and members have an understanding of the main principles of teamwork. These can then be used to guide the development of multiprofessional teams as the overall principles can be adapted and applied to the specific needs of the team. These principles are outlined below.

THEORIES OF TEAMWORK

Theory X Theory Y

Douglas McGregor was a social psychologist whose main area of interest was the way people behaved in organisations. He argued that managers based their management approach on the assumptions they had about human nature. In large part his work was a

Managing in the wider environment

reaction against an approach called 'scientific management' (Taylor 1911) which was dominant in the early part of the 20th century. The assumptions underlying scientific management are characterised by theory X, i.e.:

> People dislike work and avoid it if possible; in order to get people to work they must be controlled, forced or threatened with punishment; they prefer to be directed and left to their own devices; they have little ambition; they are motivated mainly by money because they are worried about their security; creativity is lacking unless it is applied in developing innovative ways of bucking the organisational rules and regulations.

This is reflective of an approach to organising people based on a series of rewards and punishments. Work is broken down into measurable tasks and people are rewarded financially for achieving production targets. The managerial focus is on the individual rather than the team. Elements of this approach continue today with piecework systems of remuneration and 'production line' approaches. However, McGregor (1960) regarded it as a limited approach as it did not release the creativity and commitment that people possess. In order to demonstrate this he argued that management should be based on a set of assumptions he characterised as theory Y, which were:

> Work is necessary for the individual's growth and that if people are committed to their work objectives they will enjoy working to achieve them; they do not require controls or coercion; people will willingly take responsibility for their work, be creative and solve management problems; people are motivated to achieve their potential.

The work of McGregor is explored further in Chapter Three.

Hierarchy of needs

Another worker in this tradition was Abraham Maslow, a humanistic psychologist and behavioural scientist. He developed the notion of a 'hierarchy of needs' to describe the factors that motivate people. He argued that people have five sets of needs and as most of the needs at one level are satisfied the person moves on to the next level (see Box 2.3). The highest level of 'self-actualisation' – i.e. to become more and more what one is, to become everything one is capable of becoming (Maslow 1954) – is the pinnacle of the hierarchy.

People's needs will change according to their situation. For example, if the trust is going through a merger and there are fewer posts than staff, people will have needs at the base of the hierarchy

> **Box 2.3**   Maslow's hierarchy of needs
>
> 1. At the first level are *physiological needs* such as food, drink, shelter and sensory satisfaction.
> 2. At the second level are *safety needs* which motivate people to avoid danger. These include the need to belong to either a family/workplace, and security.
> 3. At the third level are *love needs*, i.e. the social need to have positive relationships with people and to avoid feeling lonely and rejected.
> 4. At the fourth level are *esteem needs*. These include the need to have self-respect, prestige status and appreciation from external sources and internal feelings of confidence, achievement, strength adequacy and independence.
> 5. At the fifth level is the need for *self-actualisation*, which is the desire to realise the ultimate potential of self.

related to their security and safety needs. Once they feel secure in the organisation they will be able to progress to higher levels where they seek achievement and esteem in their work. It is difficult to be creative and positive about a job of place of work if you do not know if you are going to be employed there next week.

Motivation–hygiene theory

Professor Frederick Herzberg, who was a clinical psychologist, developed the concept of 'job enrichment'. He examined factors concerning individuals' attitudes to their jobs. Herzberg found that there appeared to be a set of factors that caused workers dissatisfaction if they were not present. These are linked to the job context and environment, and *are separate from the job itself*. Herzberg termed these 'hygiene factors'. Separate to these is another group of factors that may motivate workers, that tend to be related to the

> **Box 2.4**   Motivation–hygiene theory
>
> | Motivator factors | Hygiene factors |
> |---|---|
> | Achievement | How people are treated at work |
> | Recognition for achievement | Salary |
> | Interesting work | Supervision |
> | Increased responsibility | Working conditions |
> | Growth at work | |

job itself. Herzberg terms these factors 'motivators'. Some examples are listed in Box 2.4

Herzberg pointed out that absence of *dissatisfaction* does not imply satisfaction, but merely the absence of dissatisfaction. Hygiene factors may exist with or without the presence of motivators, and motivators may exist alongside dissatisfaction. Herzberg believes that managers should strive to ensure the presence of hygiene factors, and to facilitate the presence of motivators to get the best out of people at work (Herzberg 1966).

Implications for teamwork

Watson (1995) characterises McGregor, Maslow and Herzberg as 'democratic humanists'. Much of what they advocate can be summarised as participation. If people are involved in determining their work and can agree on the objectives of the team they are likely to contribute more. If they feel part of something and are valued by their colleagues they will be happier at work and make an active contribution to the work of the team. These are central principles for the effective working of multiprofessional teams. It may be difficult and present numerous practical challenges; however, it is important that the team members have an opportunity to meet and discuss their work. People need to feel involved in the decisions that are taken by the team and that their contribution is recognised. Although this may appear to be a simple requirement it often needs a great deal of energy and persistence to ensure it occurs.

The three circles model

John Adair used the work of McGregor, Maslow and Herzberg in developing a model of teamwork and leadership which he represents as three interlocking circles (Fig. 2.1).

He recognised that teams can be very different but that they have three things in common:

- *Task needs* – the need to develop a new service, for example, and/or care for patients on a ward or in a practice.
- *Group maintenance needs* – the need to develop and maintain working relationships, so that the task can be achieved. For example, it is not possible to develop or deliver a service as an individual; this involves interaction with and reliance on colleagues. Consequently there is a maintenance need of the group and this may be neglected, particularly if people are busy or feel under pressure.

How to work with other professionals

43

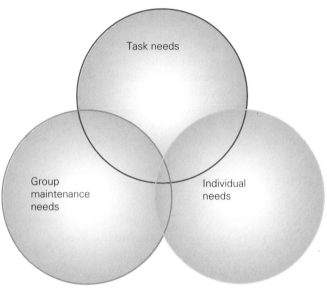

Figure 2.1 Three circles model (reproduced with kind permission from Adair 1988)

- *Individual needs* – the needs of individuals in a team such as those identified by Maslow. People come into a team with a range of individual needs which require addressing.

Implications for teamwork

Adair's (1986, 1988) work indicates that if too much attention is directed to the group or the team needs, identified by the democratic humanists, there is a risk of neglecting the task and losing sight of individual needs as people become subsumed within the team. If too much time and effort is spent on getting people to 'gel as a team' it may be that some of the work is not done. Team meetings are a good idea and a useful way of building teams; however they can be time consuming and the need for group maintenance must be balanced with the task need. Indeed if a team does not achieve its tasks it is not really effective. In addition, the reality of practice affords little 'time out' for team-building activities.

Achieving the appropriate balance between the different needs of the team is the outcome of a number of factors, one of which is effective leadership – a key component in successful teamwork. This is reflected at the policy level as the government has invested heavily in a clinical leadership strategy to develop leaders at all levels of the NHS (DoH 2000a). The role of the leader is to help and guide the team to achieve its task, to maintain the unity of the group, and to help ensure each member of the team gives of their best, and is addressed in more detail in Chapter Five. Another factor is an understanding of how people function within teams. Two areas of work provide useful insights relating to this: Belbin's work on team roles and Tuckman's model of group formation.

Belbin's team roles

Meredith Belbin is a psychologist and expert in training. Over a number of years he has examined how and why teams work and developed psychometric tests to assess individuals and their contribution to the team. This work began with studies of teams of managers at Henley Management College and was later extended to organisational teams in general. One of his conclusions was that a team made up of the brightest people did not necessarily turn out to be the best. He found that what was needed for a team to work well was the right combination of people able to fulfil eight roles that are needed in teams. The roles all have particular strengths and weaknesses which when present in the right combination complement and compensate for each other (Table 2.1).

Implications for teams

It is rarely possible to select the ideal team. Achieving the right combination, particularly in a field such as health care, is extremely difficult. For example, not only is the right combination of professional roles/functional skills needed (e.g. nurse, physiotherapist, occupational therapist, doctor, social worker, dietitian, etc.), the right blend of team roles is also needed. Multiprofessional teams often come together out of necessity rather than the team being carefully selected and developed. In addition, membership of the team changes as different groups will often send 'representatives' from another team in which they work. If the requirement is for a physiotherapist on the multiprofessional team, it could be a different physiotherapist on different occasions as the Physiotherapy Department sends a representative rather than a named individual. Similarly different nurses are likely to be members of the team depending on their availability, determined by their shift pattern. Consequently multiprofessional teams tend to have a very 'fluid' membership.

Applying the principles derived from Belbin is not possible in the sense of building the team around the identified roles. However, it is

45

Managing in the wider environment

Table 2.1 Belbin's team roles (after Belbin 1993)

Role	Strengths	Allowable weaknesses
The Chairman	Coordinates the group and has the capacity to treat all contributors on their merits Has a strong sense of objectives Usually disciplined, balanced and focused Can talk to, listen to and work through others	Ordinary intellect Not necessarily creative
The Shaper	Highly strung, dynamic and outgoing Passionate, extrovert and a spur to action Has drive and challenges inertia, ineffectiveness and complacency	Can be prone to provocation, irritation and impatience with others
The Plant	Individualistic, serious, introverted Intellectually dominant with imagination Source of original and creative ideas in the team	Can switch off if not engaged May be impractical and careless of detail
The Monitor-Evaluator	Sober, unemotional, prudent Brings an analytic dimension to the group Has sound judgement and discretion	Lacks inspiration Not able to motivate others
The Resource-Investigator	Extroverted, enthusiastic, communicative Able to bring new contacts to the team Has the ability to explore anything new and respond to challenges	May lose interest quickly May not drive the ideas forward
The Company Worker	Conservative, dutiful, predictable, methodical Good administrative/organisational skills Has practical common sense and works hard	Lacks flexibility Unresponsive to new untested ideas

Table 2.1 – *continued*		
Role	**Strengths**	**Allowable weaknesses**
The Team Worker	Socially oriented, enthusiastic and understanding Able to respond to people and situations, thus fostering team spirit	Indecisiveness at moments of crisis Can lose sight of the task
The Completer-Finisher	Painstaking, orderly, conscientious Has ability to follow a task through Pays attention to detail/seeks perfection in the attention to detail	Tendency to worry about small details Reluctance to recognise a task is complete

possible for team members to be aware of the roles they play and to adjust these as necessary. Most people do not play just one of the roles. It is possible to assume different roles in different settings and to take on more than one role. So, for example, if your preferred role is monitor-evaluator, this could conceivably be a basis for acting as a completer-finisher as well. In this way two team roles are brought together in the person of one individual along with that person's professional expertise and input. The notion of Belbin's team roles can be used to assist in the organisation of the work of the team by ensuring that work tasks are allocated appropriately among the team members. For example, if there is a particularly complex set of physical and social needs which are affecting the discharge of a patient, the resource-investigator would be able to respond to a creative solution proposed by the plant, which would then be followed up by the completer-finisher once its feasibility had been examined by the monitor-evaluator.

It is also useful to bear in mind that if there are too many people taking on the same role in a team it is unlikely to be a productive one. Again this insight can be used to understand why the team is not functioning and to encourage people to consciously take on other roles to ensure the tasks are completed.

One of the ways issues of this kind are resolved is through the interaction generated when the team is working together and developing. Once again, however, this is not a straightforward process. Some teams come together and work well from the start, others take some time, and yet others never manage to work productively and cooperatively. Some of the reasons for this have already been alluded to, such as lack of agreement on goals,

How to work with other professionals

different priorities arising from different perspectives on patient need and incompatible team roles. A useful way of highlighting the issues involved in group formation is to use Tuckman's model.

The stages of group formation (Tuckman)

Tuckman (1965) found that a group goes through various stages before it performs to its potential, if indeed it ever reaches this stage. People have to get to know each other and an atmosphere of trust and openness is needed if teamwork is to occur. When the group has formed members can discuss sensitive issues without fear of ridicule, and conflict and disagreement can be handled positively. Groups and teams change and are dynamic and sometimes this can be unsettling for the members.

The four stages in a group's development have been described as:

1. *Forming* – this is when the group first comes together. There is often anxiety surrounding the task and the purpose of the group. Members are uncertain as to what is acceptable behaviour and there is little sharing of information between people. Trust is minimal.

2. *Storming* – this is the conflict stage where issues are discussed and questions are asked. Tensions can arise as each group member's real views and beliefs come to the surface. If well handled at this stage this agreement and debate can result in the group becoming more realistic and resolve potential conflicts early on. It can be an unsettling and disruptive process but is necessary for the group members to develop trust and determine their place.

3. *Norming* – this is when the group begins to reach agreement on how it will work, how decisions will be made, and what degree of trust and openness is appropriate. This may involve 'agreeing to disagree' on some issues whilst resolving others.

4. *Performing* – When the three stages above have been completed successfully the group will begin to function to its potential.

Implications for teamwork

A team is a group of people coming together to carry out specific activities. Teams are human enterprises. Bringing people together, or allocating people to a multiprofessional team does not automatically ensure that teamwork will occur. The stages of group formation described by Tuckman (1965) can be traumatic for some individuals and result in them having a negative view of teamwork.

A fundamental point is that teamwork is founded on trust. This takes time to develop. If teams have transient members, if the focus of the work keeps changing or if there is a lack of leadership it is not surprising that teamwork in its ideal form is a rarity. In addition, the dual lines of accountability noted earlier can create problems of loyalty and focus. However, the knowledge of the challenges involved and the recognition that it is acceptable not to achieve the 'ideal' can provide a basis for progress. The principles derived from the literature indicate what should be aspired to, not necessarily what is achievable. If expectations are set too high, disappointment and disillusionment can soon follow. The principles need to be used as guidelines for best practice and applied in the real setting.

People do not usually neatly mirror the team roles and when you are in a team or a group which is not functioning it is not easy to view it as dispassionately as going through stage 2 of Tuckman, because you are living through it and experiencing the associated confusion and distress. However, it is important to persist. The alternative is to capitulate and although effective teams, in terms of the literature, are rare they do exist. Working as part of a team is a satisfying and rewarding experience and, as was mentioned at the beginning of this chapter, effective teams save lives. This is why it is an aim worth pursuing. If this is to be achieved it is necessary to examine the particular features of multidisciplinary teams. The principles discussed thus far are general to all teams. In the next section work which has been conducted on multiprofessional teams is presented as this needs to be taken into account along with the general principles as a means of fostering teamwork in the NHS.

THREE TYPES OF MULTIPROFESSIONAL WORKING

As part of a 3-year research study into multiprofessional working and shared learning Miller et al (2001) conducted in-depth case studies of six multiprofessional teams in a range of specialisms. As a result of their work they identified three main types of interprofessional working: integrated, fragmented and core, and periphery. They found that there are a variety of team structures and ways of working in the NHS.

Integrated working

This type of working existed in an organisational context of stability and predictability. This enabled the team to plan its work and to

How to work with other professionals

develop a detailed knowledge of colleagues and patients. It tended to occur where professionals were designated to a particular specialism and did not have extensive demands on their time from other teams. This situation fostered the development of team allegiance and group identity. These teams served the same population of patients and so there was a clear focus for the work and an identity for the team associated with the specialism.

This resulted in a joint approach to the organisation of the team based on collaborative meetings, shared care planning and evaluation of care. This way of working involved openness in communication, with team members being encouraged to raise issues about patients and professional concerns. Team practice remained dynamic because challenge to the status quo was encouraged by facilitative leadership in the context of a strong, safe learning environment. Central to this way of working was the development of professional skills and knowledge by team members. It was found that teams operating in this way brought several benefits to patients including:

● continuity of care
● consistency and a reduction of ambiguity in information given to patients
● appropriate and timely referral because team members understood each other's role and knew when to refer a patient to another member of the team
● actions and decisions were based on both a holistic and a problem-solving approach.

Interestingly in the research only one example of this type of team was reported. It was a neuro-rehabilitation team which was based in a purpose-built, 20 bed unit caring for patients who were medically stable. Although even within this setting there were still some rifts and problems, in many ways it represents the ideal conditions for interprofessional working. It indicates that interprofessional working can occur and that benefits can accrue when the setting and focus are 'right'. However, in many instances such ideal conditions are not present.

Fragmented working

This is illustrated by the second type of multiprofessional working discovered by Miller et al (2001) which they termed fragmented working. The teams' management of patient care in the areas of problem solving and decision making was driven by the actions of single-profession groups. Partly as a result of this, communication

Managing in the wider environment

between team members was brief and centred on giving information, rather than sharing of professional perspectives. Consequently role understanding was superficial and role boundaries were actively protected, thus reinforcing the monoprofessional nature of practice. This is an example of the 'tribalism' referred to in the English National Board report noted earlier. When professions operate in a 'tribal' way the concern is more with the needs of the professional group rather than the needs of the patients.

Leadership tended be problematic in fragmented teams because the leaders were either autocratic and took decisions without consulting staff, or they steered decision making without consensus. This created an environment where communication and learning were difficult to achieve.

In contrast to the integrated team, there was lack of awareness of the benefits to patients that could be achieved through collaboration. The teams did not discuss how effective teamwork could be achieved and so did not reach agreement on how to operate as a team. This meant the potential benefits of working in this way were not realised.

Core and periphery working

The third form of multiprofessional working that Miller et al discovered was core and periphery, which incorporated features of both integrated and fragmented working within the team. These teams tended to have a core group, which worked in an integrated way, whilst the remainder of the team was peripheral to the core and functioned in a fragmented way. The dislocation of the peripheral group from the core had an adverse effect on communication between the two groups. This also contributed to a lack of understanding of others' roles.

This type of working can be the outcome of the growth of a team in which the original members know each other well and have established effective ways of working. This arrangement continues as new members join the team resulting in the exclusion of the new members from the core group. Another contributory factor is when the roles of the team members were such that they were also involved with other teams which led to them not being regarded as 'core members' of the multiprofessional team.

Miller et al (2001) conclude that although integrated working is the most effective way of providing care for patients, regarding it as a 'yardstick' for multiprofessional working may ultimately be self-defeating. The circumstances necessary to achieve this in its 'pure form' are seldom in place and if working in this way is

How to work with other professionals

presented as what practitioners should aspire to, it could lead to demoralisation. Miller et al suggest that their work be used as a basis for discussion and reflection on the nature of multiprofessional teamwork in order to assist team members in developing appropriate approaches for their own teams. This course of action is also recommended by Øvretveit (1997), who outlines how approaches to conceptualising interprofessional working can aid practitioners. These approaches can be used to:

- plan and design the best type of team for a particular population or service
- enable teams to clarify how they are organised and the choices open to them in the future
- enable managers to understand and review the teams for which they are responsible.

FUNCTIONING OF MULTIPROFESSIONAL TEAMS

Øvretveit (1997) has investigated the way that multiprofessional teams function and, based on this work, has developed four ways of describing and defining teams. The terms he advocates are: integration, team membership, team process and team management.

Integration

This refers to the degree of integration that exists within a multi-disciplinary team. Øvretveit (1997) maintains that the best way to think of this is by means of a continuum of 'degree of integration'. At one end of the continuum is a loose-knit team called a 'network', which some would not actually regard as a team because its membership changes frequently and it is voluntary. At the other end of the continuum is a closely integrated team where the members' workload and clinical decisions are governed by a team policy and decisions made at team meetings. This continuum accounts for much of the experience of 'closeness' of interprofessional working. The location of the team, in terms of this continuum, will affect the experience of those working in the team and the type of service it provides. This is influenced by whether or not the team is formally constituted to serve a defined population or whether it is a 'looser' group that comes together as the need arises. Additionally, the degree of collective responsibility felt by the team will determine

Managing in the wider environment

its location on the continuum. Clearly structural matters are also important here in that the way the team is established in the first place is a crucial factor in terms of where it sits on the continuum.

Team membership

Membership defines a group's boundaries and often becomes an issue as teams develop. Clarifying membership tends to mark the transition from an informal loose-knit group to a more formal and organised team and this generally happens as a result of building a clearer agreement as to the purpose of the group. This involves the assignment of different categories of membership, often differentiating 'core' and 'associate' members, dependent on their function and contribution. This process can also entail taking decisions on the skill mix needed within the team to meet the demands made by client needs. Conversely, team membership is often the result of historic staffing decisions.

The other element that Øvretveit (1997) believes it is important to consider in this area is the specific skill levels of each individual member and the contribution made to the team's work. The extent to which the team is comfortable with and able to discuss differences between team members, in terms of status and function, will also affect the way the team operates.

Team process

This aspect of interprofessional working is concerned with how teams make decisions about a patient's 'journey' through the health care system. Øvretveit identified six common types of team process which can be used to identify differences in the way teams work. These range from parallel pathway teams in which each profession has its own pathway and team meetings are for the purpose of referring patients across onto other pathways, through to reception–assessment–allocation–review teams where an integrated team-based approach is taken in arriving at decisions about treatment and care.

Team management

Øvretveit (1997) utilises five main categories of team management structure:

- General management
- Profession management

How to work with other professionals

53

- Joint management
- Contracted-profession managed
- Hybrid managed.

Each of these is described in detail, and readers might wish to examine the original text for more detail.

Øvretveit clearly indicates two key challenges to be considered when identifying structures of multidisciplinary teams:

1. Establishing management structures that allow appropriate autonomy for different professionals with differing levels of seniority.
2. Establishing responsibility for managing the total resources of the team, including assessing clinical need and ensuring that practitioners' time is allocated to areas where demand is most pressing.

The complexity of the decision-making process to achieve this must not be underestimated. Complexity arises in part by the differing values and cultures of the team of established professionals, and can become even more complex as new roles are developed. When establishing a multidisciplinary team eight key tasks of individual accountability are seen to be important:

1. Drafting the job description.
2. Interviewing and appointing.
3. Introducing the person to the job.
4. Assigning work (holding accountable).
5. Reviewing work (holding accountable).
6. Annual performance appraisal and objectives-setting.
7. Ensuring practice quality, training and professional development.
8. Disciplinary action.

It is interesting that Øvretveit does not discuss in detail the issue of accountability for the shared team approach.

A final point to consider in multidisciplinary team management is the allocation of supervisors. Øvretveit cites anecdotal evidence that inadequate supervision by staff not fully aware of the demands of the professional role leads to lower quality, higher turnover and absenteeism and sickness.

This method of describing and defining teams further underlines the complex nature of such teams and the diverse issues that have to be taken into account if such teams are to function effectively. In the final part of the chapter some overall conclusions about interprofessional teamwork are presented, along with a

Managing in the wider environment

suggestion of how health care workers may have to approach teamwork in the future.

CONCLUSIONS

The principles of teamwork examined in this chapter suggest that in all teams members need to be clear about:

- their roles and responsibilities
- the task the team is trying to achieve
- how they are going to be achieved
- the indicators that will be used to judge success.

This requires effective leadership and an understanding of the dynamics of teamworking. It is important that the team is motivated. There needs to be a level of interdependence. Team members' involvement should arise out of commitment to the work of the team and a reliance on other members in order to achieve its outcomes. This results from working on important problems in which each person has a stake. Ideally there should be opportunities for reflexivity when team members reflect upon the team's objectives, strategies and processes, as well as their place in the wider organisation and environments, in order to adapt their approach as necessary. In the present health care climate this may be difficult to achieve for some of the reasons outlined earlier; however, the need for teamwork is so important that it must remain a concern for all health workers. Many of the principles of effective teamwork have been known for some time, yet the challenges to teamwork often prevent their observance. One way of overcoming this is to think constantly of new ways of applying sound principles and adapting teamwork to changing environments. An example of this is presented below.

The dolphin approach to teamwork

There is a need to develop different ways of working to be responsive to the new NHS agenda. In their book *The Strategy of the Dolphin*, Lynch & Kordis (1990) explain how dolphins use teamwork to survive the potentially fatal challenge of a shark attack. Although the shark is the ultimate predator, dolphins can be deadly to sharks. They can kill a shark by working as a team. They circle and butt the shark with their bulbous noses until the shark's ribs are crushed and it sinks to the bottom. Once it is immobile it cannot 'breathe' and dies. Dolphins are able to do this because they are adaptable, can negotiate and be proactive. They can work as team players and if things do not work one way, they change tactics until something does work. Dolphins work and think collaboratively. In this way the team is able to overcome a seemingly intractable problem – a useful approach for all health care professionals if they are to adapt to the changes in health care.

Discussion questions

- What are the differences between multiprofessional, interprofessional and interdisciplinary teamworking?
- What do you see as the barriers to effective teamworking? How can you remove some of these barriers to effective teamworking in your workplace?
- In what ways may collaborative teamwork benefit patient care?
- Does the team of which you are a member conform to Belbin's concept of team roles, and if so, what part(s) do you see yourself as playing?
- How might patients be made to feel part of the team?

References

Adair J 1986 Effective teambuilding. Gower, Aldershot

Adair J 1988 Effective leadership. Pan Books, London

Belbin M 1993 Management teams: why they succeed or fail. Butterworth-Heinemann, London

Borrill C, West M, Dawson J, Shapiro D, Rees A, Richards A, Garrod, Cartetta J, Carter A 2001 Team working and effectiveness in health care. Aston University, Birmingham

Carter A J, West M A 1999 Sharing the burden: team work in a health care setting. In: Firth-Cozens J, Payne R L (eds) Stress in health professionals: psychological and organizational causes and interventions. Wiley, Chichester, p 191–202

Davis C 1988 Philosophical foundations of interdisciplinarity in caring for the elderly, or the willingness to change your mind. Physiotherapy Practice 4: 23–25

Department of Health 1996a Primary care: delivering the future (96/395). HMSO, London

Department of Health 1996b The NHS: a service with ambitions (Cm 3425). HMSO, London

Managing in the wider environment

Department of Health 1996c Primary care: choice and opportunity. HMSO, London

Department of Health 2000a The NHS plan: a plan for investment, a plan for reform. Department of Health, London

Department of Health 2000b Improving working lives. Department of Health, London

Department of Health 2001 Investment and reform for NHS staff – taking forward the NHS plan. Department of Health, London

English National Board for Nursing, Midwifery and Health Visiting 1997 Preparation for multi-professional/multiagency health care practice. The nursing contribution to rehabilitation within the multi-disciplinary team: literature review and curriculum analysis. ENB, London

Firth-Cozens J 2001 Multidisciplinary teamwork: the good, bad and everything in between. Quality in Health Care 10(2): 65–66

Herzberg F 1966 Work and the nature of man. World Publishing, Cleveland

Leathard A (ed.) 1994 Inter-professional developments in Britain: an overview. In: Going inter-professional: working together for health and welfare. Routledge, London, p. 3–37

Lynch D, Kordis P 1990 The strategy of the dolphin. Ballantine Books, New York

Martin V, Henderson E 2001 Managing in health and social care. Routledge, London

Maslow A 1954 Motivation and personality. Harper and Row, New York

McCallin A 2001 Interdisciplinary practice – a matter of teamwork: an integrated literature review. Journal of Clinical Nursing 10: 419–428

McGregor D C 1960 The human side of enterprise. McGraw-Hill, New York

Miller C, Freeman M, Ross N 2001 Interprofessional practice in health and social care. Arnold, London

Mullins L J 2002 Management and organisational behaviour, 6th edn. Prentice Hall, Harlow

Øvretveit J 1993 Coordinating community care – multidisciplinary teams and care management. Open University Press, Buckingham

Øvretveit J 1997 How to describe interprofessional working. In: Øvretveit J, Mathias P, Thompson T (eds) Interprofessional working for health and social care. Macmillan, Houndmills, p 9–33

Taylor F W 1911 The principles of scientific management. Harper, New York

Tuckman B W 1965 Development sequence in small groups. Psychological Bulletin 63: 384–399

Watson T J 1995 The sociology of work and industry. Routledge, London

West M 2002 The HR factor. Health Management 6(6): 13–14

How to work with other professionals

Application 2:1
Anna Houston and Jeanette Clifton

A case study on consensus management:
the story of developing a corporate caseload in health visiting

In this application, Houston and Clifton present a fascinating case study which outlines a project carried out by a group of health visitors. They report not only on the hands-on care element of delivering the project, but also on the underpinning theory that informed their work.

INTRODUCTION

Historically health visitors have worked with individual caseloads of families. Sometimes their work has been based on a geographical patch or defined according to a general practice caseload. This has led to a sense of discontent when the work was unevenly distributed, with some health visitors having larger caseloads than others. The inequity of work division and concerns over child protection cases led to new ways of working such as shared caseloads and teamwork.

In West Sussex in 1997 a small group of health visitors decided to change their individual caseloads to a joint caseload in an effort to distribute work more evenly, provide an equitable service to clients and gain time to initiate public health work. Different types of corporate working existed prior to the development of this model (Rowe 1989, 1991, Gastrill 1994, Jackson 1994, Bull et al 1995, Ferguson 1996) and included different types of caseload management (Walls & Daniel 1996).

A pilot project was started, with the support of senior and middle management, to develop a new way of working. The health visitors were all female, experienced and had shown commitment to practice through their involvement in a variety of projects and policy changes within their health trust. Individual practitioners felt they had areas of expertise and knowledge that were not fully utilised. The philosophy of corporate working was researched and considered appropriate in this situation. Time was allocated for the change process and management assisted during the difficult time of moving from individual caseloads to a shared way of working. It was vital to have management support at this time because the impact of the change in service delivery affected not only health practitioners, but also clients and other external organisations. Service and organisational change was agreed when new health visitors were employed within the team.

FIRST STEPS

The first steps in developing a corporate caseload included reorganising the case files held for each family (1000 records). These case notes were centralised and filed alphabetically (the former individual health visitor systems were not conducive to the new way of working). It was vital that information, in all forms, could be accessed easily, efficiently and simply by all team members. The cooperation of clerical staff, reception staff and colleagues was also important if the new system was to be a success and misunderstandings avoided.

Creating new systems meant sharing:

- a large birth ledger
- a communications/message and referrals book
- well-baby clinic duties
- child development assessment duties on a rota basis.

It also meant sharing physical space differently, so desks, chairs, filing cabinets and storage systems were all moved.

At this time emotional energy was high. This caused stress, anxiety, uncertainty, excitement and enthusiasm.

Issues of professional accountability had to be considered. Working as a team meant agreements such as 'named health visitors' for child protection work, as well as actively considering continuity of care (Swain 1999). As well as supporting and providing guidance on these issues, the Nursing and Midwifery Council (NMC) *Code of Professional Conduct* summarises professional accountability as:

> **4.5** When working as a member of a team, you remain accountable for your professional conduct, any care you provide and any omission on your part. (NMC 2002)

Health visiting is a complex activity involving both giving and receiving in a personal interaction with clients (Luker & Chalmers 1990, Cowley 1991, 1995, Pearson 1991, Cameron 1992, Chalmers 1992, 1994, de la Cuesta 1993), an activity that can be both satisfying and challenging. In order to interact with clients in the help, advice,

A case study on consensus management

59

reassurance and support role highlighted by Machen (1996), it must be recognised that continuity of support is essential. However, too much involvement can be dangerous to both client and professional (Dale et al 1986, NMC 2002). Health visitors in the new team were willing to share the load and also to let go of previously held responsibilities (e.g. families with whom a long-term relationship had been developed). In the early months some of the readjusting was a difficult process.

UNEXPECTED SPIN-OFFS FROM CORPORATE WORKING

Potential positive aspects

Filing case records centrally and sharing everything allowed individual practice to become more open to scrutiny and group reflection. This was regarded as a positive action allowing clinical governance issues within the team to be addressed:

> Clinical governance is about creating systems that ensure safe and effective clinical practice at both an organisational and an individual level, bringing together all previously existing activities which contribute to quality improvement, for example quality standards, clinical effectiveness, research and development, education and training and risk management. (Houston et al 2001)

Potential negative aspects

Many of the actions taken by experienced health visitors in the practice were justified through 'knowing in practice' (Eraut 1994). However, vigilance and awareness of the 'dangerousness' that can develop in community practice (Dale et al 1986) were necessary. Special consideration was given, in this new corporate way of working, to the potential of developing negative 'group think' with long-term families in the new shared care method. The concept of 'group think' is described in Chapter Three. Regular discussion and corporate reappraisal were needed to avoid this aspect of sharing.

A mixed team of both full-time and part-time health visitors meant that fresh perspectives were always being introduced; maintaining the new dynamism in practice required intensive communication between team members.

COMMUNICATION WITH CLIENTS AND COLLEAGUES

Initially families had to be reminded that any member of the team could be accessed. The old way of 'owning' 'my health visitor' was altered and feedback from families demonstrated that most had no difficulty in working with the team approach. 'Packages of care' were developed to meet the commissioning requirements of the new system (Merrington 1997). These 'packages' were agreed with individual families for periods of time and this method enhanced the 'active and passive caseload' development that was so important to the new model. Those families visited regularly for whatever reason were aware that support was offered for a defined time with a purpose. A family assessment tool – the Field of Words (Houston & Cowley 2002) – was developed to use with families to assist the process of uncovering need. A contract of visits was then agreed and professional boundaries defined.

Both clients and professional colleagues in other disciplines had to be informed of this new way of working. Health visitors would not 'just pop in' to see how things were going. Working as a team helped to liberate the health visitors from the view that the role of the health visitor was to 'soft police' families or visit without a reason. Learning to trust a colleague to offer advice and perhaps visit a family previously visited 'exclusively' by you required a change in attitude and an acceptance that the work was more important than individual egos and sensibilities.

Communication within the team was essential to continue the sharing process (Hargie et al 1987). A 2-hour weekly meeting to allocate work and update each other was necessary. Attendance at this meeting was 'set in stone' because of the importance of allocating, reflecting and discussing work within the team. Consideration and discussion of referrals was also part of this forum, as was planning of group work and future community development. Passionate discussion, listening and reflection became essential elements (Schon 1991) of the weekly meetings which were tightly structured, a principle held to as a discipline in corporate working (Pedler et al 1991).

Gradually the casework changed from 'my families' to 'our families', requiring the best possible service we could provide. The team developed knowledge and acceptance of each other's strengths and weaknesses, and discovered that working together avoided the pitfalls of collusion, manipulation and 'burn-out' with families, as highlighted by Dale et al (1986).

Confidence was gained in using the wealth of expertise that existed within the team. Areas of weakness or inexperience – now apparent in 'open working' – were tolerated, and supportive learning was encouraged.

4.2 You are expected to work corporately within teams and to respect the skills, expertise and contributions of your colleagues.
(NMC 2002)

To challenge and yet encourage colleagues is not easy to master, particularly for health visitors socialised within a hierarchical nursing structure. However, corporate working offered an opportunity to

A case study on consensus management

develop practice, to admit mistakes, and to seek support when emotional reserves were low and go home, knowing that you were not the only health visitor able to respond to a situation. The burden was no longer one to be carried alone, but a shared experience both emotionally and psychologically.

WORKING WITH OTHERS

Working corporately does not mean working in a closed environment. All members of the primary health care team respond and interact with health visitors. An educative process was required to inform GPs, the mental health team and community midwives, as well as social services, of the changes made to service provision. This stage was difficult because people prefer a named person to refer to when making links to a service.

The time-consuming work of short reports to health visiting management was also important in communicating the change. Support staff such as clerical workers, receptionists and post room staff are important people in every organisation and are often excluded in change consultation. Eventually, key people who really needed new information about the service change (e.g. duty lists) were identified and information was given to them on a weekly basis. Corporate working was an opportunity to consider why we give information to some people and not to others.

STATISTICS AND GROUP WORK

Sharing information became a great strength of corporate working. Individual birth books gave way to the collective. New areas of need came to the fore developed from central statistics – for example, a higher than national average number of teenage pregnancies, a higher than national average number of postnatally depressed women. There was also an increase in the refugee population, in line with the government aim of distribution of asylum seekers outwith London. All of this 'pooled' information provided evidence for further resource and more change within the system.

As a result of working collectively, group work became focused on areas of need, highlighted through statistical analysis and the process of evaluation and re-evaluation. Public health work became possible because staff were free to share commitments and responsibilities. The team also found that they could release and support an individual member working on a cause (e.g. the support and language group developed for Kurdish families).

Expertise within the team was developed, and a need that was uncovered could be championed (e.g. a support group for women

Managing in the wider environment

experiencing postnatal depression was instituted). This is an example of 'joined up working' as suggested by Mackerith (1999).

EVALUATION

This way of working began as a pilot project and grew into normal provision. Continual evaluation and reflection on the process was essential. Keiffer (1984) called this 'praxis' and suggested it was the circular relationship of experience and reflection that allowed the development of new understanding and provoked more effective action. This explanation fitted well with the type of listening, changing evaluation and re-evaluation that was undertaken in this new way of working (Houston & Clifton 2001).

Protected time, in the form of 'away days', one each year since the inception in 1997, were used to critically appraise the past year's work and the next year's objectives. Management supported these days and attended for health visiting findings on specific subjects.

Roles that became important in corporate working included that of 'G' grade health visitors as managers as highlighted in Table 2.1.1.

Evaluation showed that what the health visitor required from line management to manage complex change included:

- support
- availability/time to discuss issues and problems
- permission to 'not get it right first time'
- a 'no blame' culture where the idea of learning from mistakes was fostered rather than scapegoating after the fact.

Benefits of collective working encompassed:

- increased level of innovation
- increased support in the workplace
- reduction of workload stress
- ability to take up different roles due to the sharing of the workload (e.g. community development)
- increased job satisfaction
- ability to implement multilayered change.

CONCLUSIONS

In this short case study we have shown how the health visitor can work corporately and still undertake effective management responsibility for caseload, clients, support staff and interagency work. We have highlighted the importance of the health visitor's own line management in facilitating this difficult process. Although working collaboratively is a tremendous challenge as highlighted by Ferguson (1996), we have shown some of the benefits of collective

A case study on consensus management

Managing in the wider environment

Table 2.1.1 Facets of the role of the health visitor in corporate working

	Working as a manager	Working as a team member	Working in partnership with colleagues and clients
Workload	Small number of specified (priority) families (40–60) with an assessed care plan Large number of normal families receiving minimal 'core' input (900+)	Working with corporate team towards caring for the large number of normal families receiving the 'core' service Sharing the care offered to the priority families	Working with families toward empowering them to resolve issues for themselves Developing trusting relationship with colleagues
Responsibilities	To other professional staff in the team: clerical assistant, nursery nurse, general nurse	To develop protocols that are robust within the team with a view to standardisation of information output from the team, e.g. all members give same information on sleep management	To clients to define the care offered Set aims and goals that the family can understand Work in an open and honest way with clients
Skills	Time management Listening ear Communicating with others Project development Dissemination of evidence-based practice	Interpersonal relationships Availability to others to allow supportive working relationships to develop	Understand the nature of consensus (Iannello 1992) Understand the nature of conflict in teams and how gender differences impact on how conflict is dealt with (Valentine 1995)

working within a motivated self-managed team. The unexpected benefit of peer support and learning together in developing the new service was gratifying.

Staff in the new system learned that effective management was about coping with continual change based on re-evaluating your own working processes. Staff also found that developing this new way of working was a challenge emotionally, psychologically and physically. It demanded that:

- inner resentments are dealt with when the consensus is difficult to reach
- practice is open to observation by others
- staff learn to critically appraise, in an appreciative way, what is done in the name of the health visiting service.

The team met all of these challenges and remained convinced of the value of the approach. Corporate working is a worthwhile model that can be applied to other aspects of community practice involving teamwork.

References

Bull S, Simons M, Wilkinson P 1995 Targeted health visiting: evaluation by clinical audit. Health Visitor 68(8): 331–332

Cameron S 1992 Games health visitors play: interaction on home visits. Health Visitor 65(7): 231–232

Chalmers K 1992 Giving and receiving: an empirically derived theory on health visiting practice. Journal of Advanced Nursing 17: 1317–1325

Chalmers K 1994 Difficult work: health visitors' work with clients in the community. International Journal of Nursing Studies 31(2): 168–182

Cowley S 1991 A symbolic awareness context identified through a grounded theory study of health visiting. Journal of Advanced Nursing 16: 648–656

Cowley S 1995 In health visiting the routine visit is one that has passed. Journal of Advanced Nursing 22(2): 276–284

de la Cuesta C 1993 Fringe work: peripheral work in health visiting. Sociology of Health and Illness 15(5): 667–682

Dale P, Davies M, Morrison T, Waters J 1986 Dangerous families: assessment and treatment of child abuse. Tavistock, London, p 26–50

Eraut M 1994 Developing professional knowledge and competence. Falmer Press, London

Ferguson L 1996 Sharing in practice: the corporate caseload. Health Visitor 69: 421–423

Gastrill P 1994 A team approach to health visiting. Primary Health Care 4: 10 12

Hargie O, Saunders C, Dickson D 1987 Group interaction and leadership. In: Social skills in interpersonal communication. Croom Helm, London, p 227–252

Houston A M, Clifton J 2001 Corporate working in health visiting: a concept analysis. Journal of Advanced Nursing 34(3): 356–366

A case study on consensus management

Houston A M, Cowley S 2002 An empowerment approach to needs assessment in health visiting practice. Journal of Clinical Nursing 11(5): 640

Houston A, Hanafin S, Cowley S 2001 What quality standards do community trusts in London need for purposes of clinical governance? NHS London Region. King's College, London

Iannello K P 1992 Decisions without hierarchy. Routledge, New York

Jackson C 1994 Strelley: teamworking for health. Health Visitor 67(1): 28–29

Keiffer C 1984 Citizen empowerment. Prevention in Human Services 3: 9–36

Luker K, Chalmers K 1990 Gaining access to clients: the case of health visiting. Journal of Advanced Nursing 15: 74–82

Machen I 1996 The relevance of health visiting policy to contemporary mothers. Journal of Advanced Nursing 24: 350–356

Mackerith C 1999 Joined up working: community development in primary health care. Community Practitioners and Health Visitors Association. College Hill Press, London

Merrington B 1997 Mid Sussex Primary Care Trust: priorities of care. Princess Royal Hospital, Haywards Heath, West Sussex

Nursing and Midwifery Council 2002 Code of professional conduct. www.nmc-uk.org/cms/content/home/home.asp

Pearson P 1991 Clients' perceptions: the use of case studies in developing theory. Journal of Advanced Nursing 16: 521–528

Pedler M, Burgoyne J, Boydell T 1991 The learning company: a strategy for sustainable development. Breaking patterns. McGraw Hill, New York, p 127–128

Rowe J 1989 Team health visiting. Hillingdon Community Health, London (unpublished papers)

Rowe J 1991 Shared caseloads and workloads. HVA Centre Circular CS 91 38

Schon D 1991 The reflective practitioner: how professionals think in action. Arena/Ashgate, Aldershot

Swain G 1999 Keeping the record straight. Community Practitioners and Health Visitors Association. College Hill Press, London

United Kingdom Central Council for Nursing, Midwifery and Health Visiting 1992 Code of professional conduct. UKCC, London

Valentine P E B 1995 Management of conflict: do nurses/women handle it differently? Journal of Advanced Nursing 22: 142–149

Walls A, Daniel K 1996 Developing an active caseload: a change in thinking. Health Visitor 69(12): 501–502

Managing in the working environment

In this application Burgess draws on her experience of leading others to provide some useful ideas for other leaders and managers when working with and developing their teams.

INTRODUCTION

The aim of this application is to help clinical managers influence their working environment by using supportive and facilitative approaches that enable their team to provide the best possible standards of care. Practical proposals to the key issues, based on experience, are suggested. Although it is recognised that others will have their own ideas, considering some of these proposals could help improve the aspects of your role as an effective clinical leader. Consequently, this could help support the team, reduce personal stress levels and improve patient care.

THE IMAGE OF THE CLINICAL MANAGER – MAKING AN IMPACT

The newly appointed clinical manager, when new to an organisation, is in a privileged position. There is the opportunity to decide on the image to be projected to others in a way that is consistent with what it is desired to achieve.

Some of the issues for the manager to consider are:

- How am I going to present myself?
- What are the personal boundaries that I am prepared to work within?
- How am I going to work?
- What can I expect from others in the form of behaviour and work?
- What will I say no to?
- How will I say no?
- What communications channels will I introduce?

● What hours will I work?
● What will I delegate?
● What image will this convey to the team?

AGREEING THE CLINICAL MANAGER'S OBJECTIVES

The manager of a clinical area will face many conflicting demands during the working day. To be an effective clinical manager, it is important to allocate time to all aspects of the role.

It is therefore important to understand the role and the job description and through this to agree priorities. These priorities should be linked with the line manager's and wider organisational objectives. This will help to ensure that priorities are related both to other clinical staff and to the wider organisation. It is useful to agree regular review dates with the line manager so that progress against objectives can be discussed and the objectives modified if necessary. By sharing objectives with others at an early stage, plans can be agreed, areas of work identified and mutually acceptable milestones agreed. These objectives can then inform personal development plans which, when developed with team members, will help to focus on key priorities.

DEVELOPING A VISION AND LONGER TERM GOALS FOR THE CLINICAL AREA

As a clinical leader it is important to have a vision for the clinical area. In developing this vision the views of the clinical team are crucial. Other potential sources for ideas for the vision include:

● *national priorities* – for example, the National Service Framework for coronary heart disease (DoH 2000)
● *national nursing, midwifery and health visiting priorities* – such as those outlined in the nursing strategy *Making a Difference* (DoH 1999)
● *the trust's strategic plan* – for example: Is the organisation planning to build a brand new hospital to replace old buildings? How should the service be shaped in the new hospital? How will care be delivered?
● *the team vision*, which can be collected through a number of fora – staff meetings, focus groups, SWOT (strengths, weaknesses, opportunities, threats) analyses, open space events, etc.
● the clinical manager's personal vision for the service.

Collecting the information will take time and the vision is not something that can be written in a hurry. It will take time to evolve.

Having collected all the information, it needs to be shaped into a plan. One approach is to write the headings onto card and organise these into a time line, putting the 5-year goals furthest away and the early goals at the front. Once the time line has been mapped out, list the priorities for year 1, year 2, etc., then list the key milestones that need to be achieved to make the vision real. Be prepared to respond to unexpected opportunities to take the vision forward. For example, if a new role for nursing forms part of the vision, think about what the job content should be and outline the job description. There are often opportunities to bid for new funding, so if the work is already prepared the clinical manager can take advantage of the situation and submit a well thought out bid for monies.

The vision should be a live document. Every few months revisit the vision. As circumstances change (e.g. a new government policy comes out), review the vision in the light of the policy so that the vision is always up to date.

Finally, always be brave about a vision. Be innovative. Do not limit the vision because it seems too adventurous, but don't forget reality. Boundaries do need to be moved forward in nursing and often boundary shifts are the result of good ideas from clinical leaders who have had the courage of their convictions.

BE AWARE OF THE BIGGER AGENDA AND USE IT TO CREATE A LOCAL VISION

The good clinical manager can further enhance their effectiveness by understanding the key local issues and the national agenda and considering how these will affect the delivery of clinical care to patients.

The local agenda

It is quite easy to establish the local agenda. Information is given out at management briefing meetings; other useful material can be obtained from Trust newsletters and minutes from Trust board meetings.

The national agenda

The national agenda is important to the clinical team: it is shaping the future direction of health care and will directly affect the clinical team and patient care.

An effective clinical manager will be aware of the political environment and be prepared to react. This can be achieved by visiting the Department of Health website (www.doh.gov.uk) and reading the press releases. Look for policies or announcements that affect the clinical service or nursing professions. Think about the relevance to the clinical area: Are there opportunities to reshape the service? Is funding available?

Influencing the agenda

Nurses are demonstrating their ability to influence others. As a clinical manager you should take some time to consider opportunities to influence the agenda, then develop a plan so that every time one of these influencing situations arises you can:

- recognise the opportunity
- deliver the message(s) in a non-threatening and constructive way
- make sure that nursing is represented appropriately.

Always have about three points prepared that sum up the issues. Aim to deliver the three points within 2 minutes to include some discussion. Prioritise the points so that if all else fails, the most important message is delivered. Practise delivering the key messages in a number of settings.

PRIORITISING THE DAILY WORK

How is the clinical manager going to work through these objectives on a day-by-day basis to support their team effectively and work towards the agreed vision?

Prioritising working time

It is important to identify how best to use the working time available. If the role is one of ward manager, it may be appropriate to allocate a management day each week, ensuring that one is not required for clinical work on these days. It may also be appropriate (e.g. when working an early shift) for the ward manager to lead the clinical team in the morning and, in the afternoon, undertake management work.

Delegation

Delegation is important to provide development opportunities for other team members and enables one to concentrate on other aspects of the role. Delegating appropriately can help to ensure that clinical care is of a high quality. Saying 'no', however, is acceptable when asked to take on work that is not within the team's remit.

COMMUNICATION

Communication is essential to the team's success. Communication needs to be clear and should convey the message in an unambiguous manner. It is useful to think of using different ways of presenting the message, since this helps to reinforce the key points.

Options to consider when communicating with the clinical team include:

- regular team meetings with recorded notes which are available for all staff to see
- extraordinary meetings to discuss urgent or unusual situations
- communication books to ensure that all staff have access to the notes of meetings and any issues that affect the running of the clinical area.

Open space events are a good way to listen to staff, to share views and agree mutually acceptable ways forward.

Coaching team members

The effective clinical manager will be able to identify when a team member needs encouragement and assistance. Coaching may be used to develop the skills and understanding of a member of staff. It provides opportunities for planned learning under guidance and supervision, drawing on the employee's work experience and often relates to learning through current situations. The coach will listen, clarify, probe and define concerns in a systematic way, and by so doing, help to develop the employee's knowledge and confidence to handle similar situations. See Chapter Six and Table 6.2.

The wider team – involving the stakeholders

One of the key issues in communication is identifying who needs to be communicated with. Some organisations have communication strategies which will provide managers with guidance on what information needs to be reported to whom, and under what circumstances. As with all policies, it is important to obtain and read these, ensuring dissemination of the key messages to other staff as required.

It is worthwhile identifying a list of potential 'stakeholders' (see Box 2.2.1) who need to be communicated with on issues in the clinical area, particularly if change needs to take place, or if there is news to tell (remember news can be good as well as bad). This list is not exhaustive, but gives an indication of the people who may need to be considered when communicating issues or changes.

Managing in the working environment

Box 2.2.1 Potential stakeholders in the clinical area

- Patients and users and their visitors/carers
- Patient interest groups
- The direct line manager
- The professional lead (if this is a different person)
- The bed manager
- The site manager
- All nursing staff in the team
- All medical staff who access the clinical area
- Other clinical professions (e.g. physiotherapists, pharmacists, etc.)
- The ward social worker
- The link lecturer or clinical teacher
- Union representatives
- Domestic staff
- Porters
- The switchboard

CONCLUSION

This application has aimed to help clinical managers influence their working environment and reduce stress by encouraging supportive and efficient approaches to managing the clinical team. Practical solutions to the key issues have been suggested, along with ideas for implementing them.

References

Department of Health 1999 Making a difference: strengthening the nursing, midwifery and health visiting contribution to health and health care. Department of Health, London

Department of Health 2000 National Service Framework for coronary heart disease. Department of Health, London

Managing in the wider environment

Section **Two**

MANAGING AND SUPPORTING PEOPLE – A PROACTIVE APPROACH

OVERVIEW

Organisations do not have a life of their own; their life stems from the activities of the individuals that work within and in partnership with them.

A characteristic of 21st century organisations is that they are in a constant state of change, change that is fuelled by changes in society, in world economic fortunes, in opportunities and in expectations. Changes at macro levels (e.g. following the events of September 11th) can impact on every part of society; changes at micro level (e.g. following a court judgement for an individual patient) can influence the wider national (and sometimes international) agenda.

It has been suggested that because of this fast changing environment, leadership is a more appropriate approach than the more formal management one. The truth and value of this assumption to a large extent rests on the *definitions* of

Managing and supporting people

leadership and management. This section seeks to offer a proactive approach, with less concern for the detail of theoretical definitions. In large organisations, both leadership and structured management will be required so that staff can move forward through innovation, and also ensure that the daily work is carried out safely and documentation is completed accurately to ensure a robust audit trail.

To enable individuals to give of their best, it is imperative that leaders and managers develop and enact a culture and structure that supports and cherishes the contribution of the workforce, both individually and collectively. This is not merely an altruistic perspective, born of 'Pollyanna' schools of management, but a pragmatic approach to ensure that the organisation gets the best out of individuals, because they, individually and collectively, feel valued and respected. Contented staff results in a better service for the service users, and that is a quality factor.

Whilst change is constant and continuous, the collective contribution of people to an organisation remains an enduring factor, and effective leadership and change management skills are important in maintaining quality care and organisational effectiveness.

Performance management is a cousin of change management, in that it seeks to use the tried and tested processes and approaches of change management to enhance organisational performance. Within this process, the individual will be adapting and changing to organisation needs and demands, but to do this, individual change will be required. This will be most effectively achieved when positive leadership is apparent.

Effective leadership ensures that staff can adjust within the context, and thus their efforts are congruent with its demands. Managed competently and positively, in an environment of positive leadership, change should be a platform of opportunity, a stimulus to develop in new fields. Managed negatively, change can have profoundly destructive effects on individuals, and therefore on organisations. There will be times when change produces discomfort, but effective leadership should be able to ameliorate this, and present it as part of the reality of life that, viewed appropriately, has a positive outcome.

Chapter **Three**

The human aspects of organisational change

Barbara Hendry

- Transformational leadership
- Situational leadership
- Personal behaviours
- Team behaviours
- The 'grieving' process

- Change analysis – PESTELI, SWOT, FFA
- Organisational culture – formal and informal
- Planning, implementing and sustaining the change process

O V E R V I E W

In this chapter Hendry addresses the complex issues of change management and makes explicit links between effective outcomes of change, and the appropriate use of leadership and management techniques.

INTRODUCTION

The cliché 'the only constant these days is change' has become more and more true; that is why it is so surprising that change is still perceived as an 'add on' to organisational life.

Managers and leaders need to be able to initiate and respond to change in a positive and proactive way in order to lead and facilitate organisational development.

Managers/leaders who can identify opportunities add value by responding to the need of the business and its customers; however, this can be counterproductive if the manager lacks the emotional maturity necessary to be able to deal with the messy, emotional, human side of change within the formal and informal culture. 'Working the shadow side' as described by Egan (1994) becomes a required skill of an effective leader. Leaders and managers must be able to understand the informal culture of organisations and know how to work effectively with the organisation's informal relationships. Egan continues by saying that the 'special favours, the broken rules, the political promotions and the undiscussed firings that take place in nearly every organisation around the world' need to be recognised by effective leaders.

These relationships will not be part of any organisational chart or found in writing in any part of the organisation. You will know the 'informal' leaders within your own team and workplace; these people are perceived to have influence within the team and organisation. Others go to these individuals for information and guidance. This is useful if these individuals are positive and proactive and understand why change is occurring. However, it can be devastating and destructive for the team if the individual's negativity is so strong that it negates any creativity and empowerment within the team. When managed effectively, these individuals become a huge asset to the leader, the team and the organisation – they can act as agents of change.

LEADERSHIP AS A PROCESS OF CHANGE

In order to manage change effectively you need to give some thought to your leadership style as this will have an impact on the change process. The activities of leadership are considered in more detail by Cook in Chapter Five. However, as there is so much interaction and co-dependency between the processes, it is also worth mentioning it here as these processes are applied in the effective management of change.

The following need to be considered if the process of change is going to be managed effectively and efficiently. The processes and application of leadership are contextual, i.e. they must fit the circumstances and cultures in which they are functioning. There are many approaches and many variables that impact on the particular approach chosen, some of which are explored below.

Transformational leadership

There are many definitions of transformational leadership. Alvolio et al (1991) state that 'a leader will have to be more than merely a manager, a leader will need to develop followers, raise their need levels and energise them'. Transformational leadership, as suggested by Bass & Alvolio (1994), comprises four basic components:

- *Idealised influence* – the charisma of the leader, and the respect and admiration of the followers
- *Inspirational motivation* – the behaviour of the leader which provides meaning and challenge to the work of the followers
- *Intellectual stimulation* – leaders who solicit new and novel approaches for the performance of work and creative problem solutions from followers
- *Individualised consideration* – leaders who listen and give special concern to the growth and developmental needs of followers.

Burns (1978) continues by suggesting that leaders and followers raise one another to higher levels of motivation and morality and, in doing so, Tichy & Devanna (1990) suggest that transformational leadership is about change, innovation and entrepreneurship that requires ongoing learning, adopting new behaviours and searching for new ways of working in order to achieve greater efficiency and effectiveness.

Situational leadership

The theory of situational leadership was developed by Hersey et al (1996) who suggest that there is no one best leadership style.

The situational leadership model identifies behaviours of the leader which support growth and development in staff or followers – just what is needed to facilitate the processes of change. This model suggests that the leader uses one of four styles depending at what stage the follower is at with a particular task or situation.

The four styles are identified in quadrants:

- Quadrant 1 – directing style
- Quadrant 2 – coaching style
- Quadrant 3 – supporting style
- Quadrant 4 – delegating style.

The leader needs to master the four styles to be able to assess the follower's development needs and how much directive and supportive behaviour the follower requires from them as a leader (Fig. 3.1). This model is easily transferable for use in the activities of change management to move forward people's behaviour.

It is useful to remember here that the overall skill of *managing people* is an eclectic role, requiring eclectic knowledge and a variety

The human aspects of organisational change

3—Supporting	2—Coaching
The leader supports the follower towards completing the task – sharing problem solving and decision making in a facilitative way	The leader is highly directive and supervises closely – but supports and guides the follower through activities such as decision making
4—Delegating	**1—Directing**
The leader gives total responsibility to the follower for all activities, decision making and problem solving	The leader gives specific and detailed instructions, and supervises the follower closely

Figure 3.1 The four styles of the situational leadership model (adapted from Hersey et al 1996)

of approaches, so it is not surprising that the change manager uses a range of different management and leadership styles.

Change should be seen as a developmental opportunity for members of the team; in utilising the situational leadership quadrants effectively, leaders will contribute to change being a positive experience for individual members of the team, but who also will, as individuals, learn and develop from the process.

KNOW YOURSELF

You are about to initiate a change or introduce a change that has been imposed from an internal or external source – where do you start?

If you have not already done so you need to spend some time to reflect and identify your own behaviours, perceptions and beliefs. If you are to manage change effectively you need to get to know yourself and be prepared to be honest about your own views. As a manager it may be that your role requires you to manage a process of change that you as an individual are not happy about. This can become apparent to others and can compromise the effectiveness of the change. Honest self-reflection can prepare for such an eventuality.

Spending time with yourself might reveal things you would rather not see – but it is necessary to invest in yourself if you are going to maintain the positive energy required when dealing with your personal transition, the team's transition and the change itself.

Managing and supporting people

Covey (1999) talks about 'sharpening the saw' and tells the following story:

> Suppose you were to come upon someone in the woods working feverishly to saw down a tree. 'What are you doing?' you ask. 'Can't you see?' comes the impatient reply, 'I'm sawing down the tree'. 'You look exhausted!' you exclaim, 'How long have you been at it?'. 'Over five hours', he returns, 'and I'm beat! This is hard work'. 'Well, why don't you take a break for a few minutes and sharpen the saw?' you enquire, 'I'm sure it would go a lot faster'. 'I don't have time to sharpen the saw' the man says emphatically, 'I'm too busy sawing'.

A sobering thought: how many times have you worked long and hard, head down, hardly pausing for a drink or lunch? (A friend of mine was known to say lunch was a yogurt on the end of a telephone.)

Working proactively

Sharpening the saw is about preserving and enhancing the greatest asset you have – yourself! Covey (1999) believes that you are at the centre of your circle of influence. He suggests that we need to look at our own degree of proactivity and where we focus our time and energy. We may find that some of our time and energy is focused in our circle of concern – for example, some strategic issues at work, world debt. Covey suggests that concerns which have an emotional or mental involvement need to be moved within our smaller circle of influence. Proactive people focus their efforts within this circle of influence, i.e. they focus on areas they can do something about. 'Their energy is positive, enlarging and magnifying causing their circle of influence to increase' (Covey 1999).

Working reactively

Reactive people focus on the weaknesses of others and circumstances over which they have no control. They focus on 'blaming and accusing attitudes, reactive language and increased feelings of victimisation' (Covey 1999). The negative energy generated by this focus, combined with neglect in the areas that they could do something about, causes their circle of influence to shrink. Thus they are likely to be less effective at dealing with change, either for themselves or for others.

The human aspects of organisational change

Think about the times when you have been stressed:

- you start to become more reactive, withdrawn and have limited time for others and for yourself
- you start blaming and accusing others at a time when you need their support and understanding
- you need your circle of influence to remain constant or expand, not to diminish.

The four dimensions of self

So back to the woodcutter and yourself. In order to preserve and enhance the greatest asset you have which is you, you need to replenish the four dimensions of our nature – physical, mental, spiritual and social/emotional – regularly and consistently.

Physical dimension

The physical dimension is concerned with caring for the physical body, eating a healthy diet, getting sufficient rest and relaxation and exercising on a regular basis. Exercise is associated with increased self-esteem and a feeling of wellbeing, and contributes to the management of stress. This is discussed further in Chapters Seven and Eight.

Mental dimension

The mental dimension comes through exploring new concepts, gaining knowledge and continuing personal and professional development. This may involve formal education through courses but there are many other ways, such as coaching, shadowing others, reading and facilitating followers' needs.

Spiritual dimension

The spiritual dimension is private, individualistic and is the centre of your value system. People find renewal of the spirit by communicating with nature, or immersing themselves in literature or music. It draws upon the sources that uplift you in times of need.

Social/emotional dimension

The social/emotional dimension is associated with our relationships with others in every aspect of our life. Personal security and harmony come from knowing yourself, your values and your personal worth.

In knowing yourself (i.e. your personal boundaries and integrity) you will know how to renew your energy, and keep positive and proactive when managing or initiating change. One of the hardest aspects of management is introducing a change with which you do not personally agree. Whilst maintaining your integrity and values it is possible to make the transition which will enable you to nurture yourself whilst enabling others to make the transition and change.

Building trust

But what are you going to let go of? What are you going to lose and acquire in the transition: What is acceptable? What is not? Whatever the change, its effectiveness will depend upon the transition which is built on the trust which exists between the leader and the team. When people do not trust each other, progress in the process of change will be slow. If you don't believe *in*, or believe *what* your manager is saying to you, it will be difficult to communicate the message to the team you lead with any degree of congruence.

Your trustworthiness will be demonstrated by your actions: you need to do what you say you will do, actively listen to others, understand what matters to people, be honest and ask for feedback on a regular basis. Without such honesty, the process of achieving change is likely to be less effective.

Management style

It may also be useful to reflect on your preferred style of management. McGregor (1960) argued that the style of management adopted is a function of the manager's attitude towards people and their assumptions about human nature and behaviour (see also Chapter Two).

McGregor's (1960) famous theory identifies two extremes on the continuum of beliefs a manager may hold. Theory X suggests that the average person is lazy, has an inherent dislike of work, and needs to be controlled and threatened with punishment if the organisation is to achieve its objectives. Theory Y, however, suggests that most people are intrinsically motivated and will work towards the organisational goals. It is the task of managers to create conditions in which individuals satisfy their motivational needs and in which they can achieve their own goals through the goals of the organisation.

Think for a moment about which approach is likely to achieve the most effective change outcomes. If you want to read more about McGregor's management approach, you will find it in any

The human aspects of organisational change

good management text. For example, both Mullins (2002) and Cole (1996) have excellent sections which explore a range of theories of people management.

KNOW THE TEAM MEMBERS

In order to manage change effectively you are wise to know your team members and have positive working relationships with them.

Whether change is perceived as a threat or an opportunity, it can still be stressful. In addition to knowing yourself you need to know the individual members of your team.

Valery, a French poet, stated that:

Every beginning is a consequence, every beginning ends something.

Bridges (1999) continues:

So beginnings depend on endings, the problem is people don't like endings. Yet change and endings go hand in hand; change causes transition and transition starts with an ending.

So some members of the team, like yourself, are going to have to let go of something, whether that be treasured beliefs, perceptions, valued working relationships with colleagues or personal working space.

Members of the team may overreact to change from the perspectives of others; however, do not forget that being reasonable is much easier when one has little or nothing at stake! Mullins (2002) suggests that individuals may be resistant to change because of fear of the unknown, security in the past, economic implications, inconvenience, loss of freedom, habit and selective perception regarding the change itself. It is worth considering these areas when you perceive someone is being 'difficult'.

Change is constant, change is becoming more complex, change is non-stop. How often have you experienced a change being introduced and then, before it can be truly implemented, let alone evaluated, it is changed again, and possibly again. We have seen this in the NHS as a result of the changing political agenda imposing organisational change. Time and again, we see change overlapping with change. On top of this everyone has personal change issues to deal with – no wonder people are at risk of becoming stressed.

Bridges (1999) talks about the three phases of transition and change:

- ending and letting go
- neutral zone
- new beginnings.

Ending and letting go

To support staff in 'ending and letting go' you will need to communicate effectively.

Be aware of how you communicate; be conscious of your spoken word and your non-verbal communication (e.g., your facial expression, personal space, use of the environment, body movement, posture, touch and silence). Remember if what you say (with words) and what you say via non-verbal communication are not congruent, this will, at best, weaken the message, and at worst cause staff to distrust not only that message, but every other message from the same source.

Remember that you, as the manager/change agent, have had time to assimilate the change and may have started to make the internal transition required. You may have some degree of control over the change. Managers often forget that they are one step ahead of the staff and wonder why the principles of change are not accepted immediately.

One of the most important aspects of communication is active listening: listen and learn and don't argue with staff during the listening process. By listening you will show team members that you wish to gain an understanding of their points of view and concerns. By genuine listening you will start to gain people's commitment; without commitment the change will not be effective.

Expect and recognise the signs of grieving for the 'ending', whatever each member of staff perceives this to be. By knowing the individual staff members you will know who has a 'work/life balance' and those members whose life fulfils the four dimensions of life in balance, i.e. the physical, mental, spiritual and social/emotional dimensions described earlier.

Staff members grieve for the loss of the pre-existing situation. The work undertaken by Elisabeth Kübler-Ross on loss (Upton & Brooks 1995) has been shown to be applicable to organisational change. Individuals go through the process at different speeds but typically will go through six stages which include:

- *Shock* – When an individual is first informed of a major change they may be unable to take it in. They may say things like 'I just don't believe it ....'. This stage is usually short.
- *Denial* – At this stage the individual has begun to take in what has been said, but is still unable to come to terms with the change as it is still not 'real'. There may be a feeling of euphoria but this is generally short lived and is an initial way of coping

The human aspects of organisational change

with the change, when admitting the degree of loss would be too much for the individual to handle. Occasionally an individual can get stuck at this stage, unable to accept the reality of the change and make plans for the future. Individuals need to be helped through this stage.

- *Blame* – At this stage the individual has begun to recognise what is happening and to feel angry about the change. They need to find a target and someone to blame. Sometimes individuals fix the blame on someone who is not the instigator of the change as a displacement tactic; this can be a difficult time for the manager or team leader. People may express their anger directly as personal hostility or be more passive, appearing to comply with the changes, but actually sabotaging them where they can.
- *Self-blame* – At this stage people move from blaming others to blaming themselves. They may feel they have done something to bring on the change (and this is their just reward, perhaps as a punishment) or they may feel that they will never be able to work to the demands of the new situation. This can make them very frightened. People may have feelings of despair or powerlessness and may present with depression. The leader needs to work with such individuals, encouraging and supporting them.
- *Bargaining* – At this stage individuals start to adapt to the new situation, exploring the new possibilities. This is a creative and developmental phase and needs to be supported by managers.
- *Resolution* – The individual has adapted to the changed situation and it has become the new status quo. Ideally any change should be followed by a period of stability so that full adjustment can take place.

Bridges (1999) supports this process, adding that some individuals will let go at different stages, working through the emotions of anger, bargaining, anxiety, sadness, disorientation and depression, and then move forward. Some people will never let go and may become bitter. If they suppress their emotions and are taken along on the tide of change they will never get through the neutral zone and into new beginnings, as they will be unable to adjust in a psychologically healthy way. It is OK to feel bad, feel angry, etc. at the beginning, but if this loss process does not follow through and individuals 'get stuck', then dysfunctional behaviours can occur. In such circumstances, professional help (e.g. counselling) may be necessary.

Teams may fall apart if significant individuals never find a way to grieve over their loss. As a manager you need to define what has ended and what has not. Bridges (1999) suggests that endings should not just be talked about, they should be visual and memorable. Mark the ending with a party, or a photographic reminder of all the good times and a celebration of past achievements; value the past and link it with the present and the future.

As a manager you should never denigrate the past; in doing so you imply covertly that all that was achieved in the past was of no value. Confronting the individuals who are being resistant to the change is not helpful, and these individuals may take the judgements personally.

Endings occur more easily if people take some part of the past with them. By celebrating the ending you support and encourage people to let go and enter the neutral zone and ultimately the new beginnings.

Neutral zone

This is the time when mistakes happen and people are loath to take risks. The time when what was comfortable and known has ended and all too often the new systems are not working effectively. This can be perceived as negative chaos unless as a manager you are there at ground level with the staff, communicating and interpreting events. Staff are anxious and motivation falls, sickness absenteeism rises and this is the time when dynamic staff will leave the organisation if the neutral zone is not effectively managed. Bridges (1999) continues by saying that 'you need to foster a spirit of entrepreneurship amongst them'.

As the health sector is moving explicitly towards self-managed teams and the concept of a learning organisation, this is likely to be welcomed by some managers, but not by others. Those managers who adopt an autocratic style in the spirit of command and control may find this approach difficult. Using the neutral zone creatively and taking managed risks is the surest way to harness the energy and courage needed to navigate through change to the new beginnings.

If the organisation has a blame culture that punishes failure (as historically the NHS has), then people will not put their heads above the parapet more than once. It is essential that as a leader or manager of change you agree the boundaries and authority associated with any project during this time; failure to do this will compromise the effectiveness of change. As services still need to be provided in health care sectors during the time of the neutral zone (they cannot close down for annual holidays!), planning for change is essential through all three phases.

The human aspects of organisational change

85

New beginnings

Bridges (1999) separates 'starts' and 'new beginnings'. He suggests that people know there is a new start when the revised organisational chart appears, and sometimes new line managers are put into post. He explains that the transition is still happening for most people and only when people have come through the neutral zone, and are ready to make the emotional commitment to do things differently, will the new beginning commence. Beginnings need to be nurtured and will follow the individual's *internal* timing, not the action dates on the implementation chart.

As a manager or leader you also need to be aware that some people may find the neutral zone comforting: the ambiguity and the slower pace give some individuals a cover, free from deadlines and pressure. Thus some may be reluctant to leave it! New beginnings signal that life will be quickening up once more and everyone will be accountable.

In working through the three phases of transition and change, the leader or manager must:

- be consistent
- ensure some quick 'win–win' situations to symbolise the new beginning
- recognise and celebrate past achievements in a manner that is acceptable to the team
- start to embed the new ways of working within the culture.

CONTEXT FOR CHANGE

So why is this change going to happen? Has it been imposed from another source, either external or internal to the organisation? Do you have to react to the change or are you being proactive in introducing change? Have you or a member of your team identified something that requires changing and developing so that a more effective service can ultimately be provided for the service user?

Change analysis

Change can be complex and often must be multidisciplinary, working across organisational boundaries and across different sectors.

In order to identify how and why the change has become necessary it is useful to undertake a PESTELI analysis. This is a checklist

Managing and supporting people

for analysing the triggers which may have emerged from different environments. The acronym reminds us of:

- *Political factors* – There are both big and small 'p' political forces and influences that may affect the performance of, or the options open, to the organisation.
- *Economic influences* – This is the nature of the competition faced by the organisation or its services, and the financial resources available within the economy.
- *Sociological trends* – These are the demographic changes (e.g. the growing elderly population, trends in the way people work, think and live).
- *Technological innovations* – New approaches to doing new and existing things do not necessarily involve technical equipment; they can be new ways of thinking and organising. However, the introduction of improved techniques (e.g. more sophisticated anaesthetic processes) impacts on the way care is delivered.
- *Ecological factors* – The globalisation agenda and the impact of the wider ecological system of which the organisation is a part, and how it interacts with the wider world are important to consider. Issues of waste management may be included under this heading and thus may be triggers to change.
- *Legislative requirements* – Originally included under 'political', relevant legislation now requires a heading of its own. All readers will have been involved in change as a result of legislation (e.g. the introduction of the internal market in the NHS in 1991 and subsequent loss of Crown immunity).
- *Industry analysis* – This is a review of the attractiveness of the industry of which the organisation forms a part, and may thus trigger changes in organisation focus.

By undertaking a PESTELI analysis, trigger factors in the environment which impede or are supportive to the change can be analysed. In complex change the PESTELI will be different for different organisations, different parts of the organisation and different sectors.

Organisational culture

Another area to explore within the context of change is the organisational culture and how this will affect, support or restrain change. Culture will be both formal and informal and may be

The human aspects of organisational change

different in each area and level of the organisation. The anthropological origins of culture are outlined in Chapter One.

Culture is an accumulation of 'the way we do things around here'. It is the norms and beliefs developed over time and is comprised of the following factors which, according to Johnson (1992), contribute to the cultural web.

- *Stories and myths* – These are told by members of the organisation and are embedded in the daily activities. They identify important events and different personalities, usually centred around the successes, failures, heroes, villains and mavericks within the organisation.
- *Symbols* – The logos, offices, cars, language, titles and the terminology used within the organisation. When managing complex change, be sensitive to the fact that certain phrases have different meanings in different organisations.
- *Power structures* – Who are the most powerful people? Are these senior people in management positions or are they individuals who are not formally responsible for others?
- *Organisational structures* – These reflect the important relationships and activities within the organisation.
- *Control systems* – The measurement and reward systems within the organisation.
- *Rituals and routines* – Special events and behaviours associated with that department or organisation.

Formal culture

Handy (1991) describes four types of formal culture:

- club
- role
- task
- existential.

Each of these cultures is different; none is better or worse but they may be inappropriate to the context and the circumstances. Change is managed more effectively in some cultures than in others.

Club culture

In the club culture one central figure is in charge. Your relationship with this person is all important; groupthink (Janis 1972) is the norm. Groupthink occurs when the group/organisation develops within itself an illusion of invulnerability which causes excessive risk taking and loss of touch with reality. Pressure is put on individuals to conform, thus reinforcing the process of collective rationalisation: 'We must be right – we all agree!'.

Step outside what is acceptable behaviour and you may be ostracised. Change is created by changing people, i.e. literally by replacement. Disloyalty to the 'club' norms is not tolerated. Change is only achieved by persons who are perceived as being 'credible' within the organisation.

Role culture

The role culture bases its approach around the definition of the role or the job to be done. This is seen in most NHS organisations where job descriptions, policies and procedures hold the organisation together. This is excellent when tomorrow will be like yesterday, and stability and predictability are the norm, but tends to be inflexible and slow to respond to change. Change will take time to introduce and sustain. Traditionally all public sector organisations have emulated a role culture.

Task culture

The task culture is energetic and creative. Performance is judged by results and outcome. Individuals are committed, and this culture only recognises expertise. This is typical of project management and managing change through a project way of working.

Existential culture

The existential culture supports people to work independently, not interdependently. This is the only culture which exists to help people achieve *individual* purpose. The skill of the individual is the crucial asset of the organisation. Change will occur only if it produces a gain for the individual. An example of this is a group of barristers sharing Chambers.

Informal culture

In addition to the formal culture which is comprised of the formal goals, financial resources, technology, physical facilities, organisation design, surface competencies and skills, rules, regulations and the service users, Mullins (2002) discusses the 'organisational iceberg' (Fig. 3.2) which identifies the formal culture (overt aspects) as being the part of the iceberg above the waves, and the informal culture as the covert behavioural aspects which lurk below the surface.

The informal culture is comprised of attitudes, communication patterns, informal team processes, personalities, conflict, political behaviour, underlying competencies and skills. In order to manage

The human aspects of organisational change

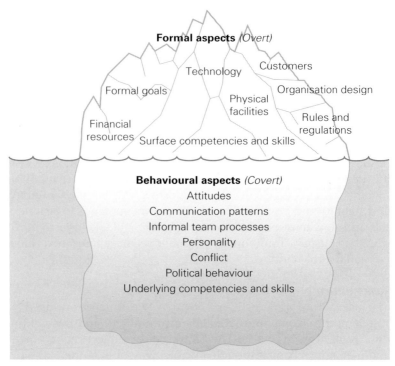

Figure 3.2 The organisational iceberg (reproduced with kind permission from Hellriegel et al 1998)

change (and therefore people) effectively, it is important that the manager is aware of, and has some understanding of, the informal culture, and also acknowledges its power.

Egan (1994) discusses the positive side of managing the covert informal culture (the 'shadow side' of the organisation) and shows how managers can develop skills for supporting a preferred culture in addition to challenging and changing a dysfunctional one. He also discusses how to deal sensitively and constructively with people's idiosyncrasies. This is vital if change is going to be effective and sustainable, and if people are to feel valued and respected.

PLANNING FOR CHANGE

When planning for change there are several tools that can assist in achieving optimal outcomes.

Change analysis

We have already discussed the PESTELI to help identify the context for change. When this has been completed a SWOT analysis (strengths, weaknesses, opportunities and threats) undertaken by the team will identify the achievements and developmental needs of the team in relation to the proposed change.

A force field analysis (FFA), as described by Lewin (1951), is a tried and tested tool which maps the assumption that in any change situation there are two sets of forces: those driving the change and those which oppose or restrain it.

It is important to recognise that these are forces as perceived by the people involved in the change. If the driving forces for change are stronger than the restraining forces it can be assumed progress will be made. Forces can be clustered under different headings (e.g. personal, organisational, technological, financial, relationships, boundary working).

To carry out a FFA, the following tasks should be undertaken:

- Identify and list forces *pushing* events to move in the right direction (driving forces).
- Identify and list forces *preventing* events moving in the right direction (restraining forces).
- Highlight the most significant of the driving and restraining forces. Which of these can you influence?
- How can you reduce or eliminate the restraining forces?

Examples of driving and restraining forces are typically demonstrated in a diagram such as the one shown in Figure 3.3.

Once you have clarity about the issues, you can then consider how the driving forces can be made more, powerful. If the

Driving forces for change	Restraining forces
management support	management capacity
policy drivers	some staff opposition
financial gain long term	lost opportunity costs short term
public support	inconvenience of building work

Figure 3.3 Force field analysis (reproduced with kind permission from Lewin 1951)

The human aspects of organisational change

magnitude of a driving force is increased, the restraining forces often respond in kind, resulting in deadlock.

Completion of the force field analysis may lead to an onset of realism. Once there is a clear view of the forces in play you need to decide what resources (e.g. time, people, information, finances, skills and knowledge) are needed to complete the change, and where you need to focus these.

In addition to the force field analysis it is useful to undertake a commitment planning exercise. Senge (1990) discusses commitment, enrolment and compliance in relation to change. It is important to identify the position of stakeholders in respect to the change, especially if individuals demonstrate non-compliance and/or grudging compliance. As the leader or manager you will need to spend time with such individuals in identifying how to enable them to move to formal and genuine compliance, reaching as far as possible a situation of fair compromise.

Lewin's model of change

Lewin's (1951) classic model of change offers a framework to manage change. He outlines three stages: unfreezing, moving and refreezing.

- In stage 1 (unfreezing) Lewin believes that the focus of energy should be on the 'undoing' of current ways of doing things so that these can become separate from the work of the organisation.
- Stage 2 (moving) is about realigning behaviours and beliefs to meet the demands required by the changes to be introduced.
- Stage 3 (refreezing) is about establishing the new 'norms' as accepted practice within the organisation.

IMPLEMENTING THE CHANGE PROCESS

Change, whether individual or institutional, is messy, emotional, social, political, cultural and counter-cultural in nature. These realities need to be factored into the change process from the very beginning. (Egan 1993)

There are several change management models. One such, entitled 'A project way of working to manage change', is based on Egan's

(1994) 'Model B' for organisational change. The steps in this change management model include:

- Proposal
- Problem analysis and diagnosis
- Developing options for change
- Producing an implementation plan
- Implementation
- Evaluating the change
- Sustaining the change.

Proposal

The proposal includes a statement of the problem or opportunity, the objective, the difference between now and then. It also includes advice on how to evaluate before, during and after the project. Achievement markers are required, such as: What milestones are appropriate to monitor the project's progress? Are they sensitive enough to deal with unexpected factors, human or otherwise? At this stage it is necessary to propose the team, membership of which is based on the ability of each member to add value to the project. A sponsorship team is useful if the manager/leader is new to managing change.

It is useful to have a team of senior staff (i.e. two to three individuals) who will act as mentors to the project team. The communication strategy – what, when, why, how and who are you to communicate with on a regular/irregular basis – also needs to be discussed and agreed.

Problem analysis and diagnosis

Identify what the real problem is utilising appropriate management tools.

Developing options for change

Have a brainstorm session identifying all the different options:

- Which options will have the most leverage?
- Which options will be most beneficial to the organisation?
- Which option would make the most positive impact on the project?
- What are the risks associated with each option?
- What is the knock-on effect (and which stakeholders will be involved) of each option?

The human aspects of organisational change

Producing an implementation plan

This is where a sequenced timed plan is agreed with an awareness of the dependencies at each step of the way. The actions are SMART, i.e. specific, measurable, achievable, realistic and time related (see Chapter Seven for another application of this process). Lead personnel are identified for each action.

It is important at this stage to include an education strategy, especially if the change involves clinical competencies. You need to consider what new skills the team requires, by whom and when the education is going to be given, and what impact this will have on the provision of the existing service (e.g. in lost opportunity costs).

Implementation

Agree a date for commencement of the changed service. The implementation plan will have identified whether this will be a 'clean break' or whether the old system will run parallel to the new system for an agreed length of time. This usually occurs when a pilot of the changed system is undertaken. It is important to know how this is going to be evaluated before a full roll out occurs. Will the team revert back to the old system during the evaluation or continue with the new system? The pilot should identify any issues that should be resolved before a full roll out occurs.

Evaluating the change

How the change will be evaluated should have been identified at the proposal stage of the change project as this needs to be factored into the implementation plan.

Sustaining the change

If the change process has been effectively managed by the leader/manager then the change will sustain itself; change is not sustained where staff have not made the transition and remain resistant to the change whatever the reason. Change which is hurried is rarely sustainable. Ongoing evaluations need to be identified within the implementation plan.

As the leader or manager of change it is useful to keep an events diary to reflect on when the change has occurred successfully and the key factors in success have been identified. This is also useful to make personal learning points for the next time for – as we said at the beginning – change is constant!

Discussion questions

- What is the leader's contribution to the management of change?
- What are the key stages of the change management process?
- How can the use of planning tools such as Lewin's force field analysis (FFA) contribute to effective change management outcomes?
- Identify a change in your workplace, or in your own life. Use the FFA tool to map out the driving and restraining forces in that change.
- How can staff be supported in seeing change as an opportunity for development rather than as a threat?

References

Alvolio B J, Waldman D A, Yammarino F J 1991 Leading in the 1990's: the four I's of transformational leadership. Journal of European Industrial Training 15: 9–16

Bass B M, Alvolio B J 1994 Improving organisational performance through transformational leadership. Sage, London

Bridges W 1999 Managing transitions – making the most of change. Nicholas Brearley, London

Burns J M 1978 Leadership. Harper and Row, New York

Cole G A 1996 Management theory and practice. Letts Educational, London

Covey S 1999 The seven habits of highly effective people. Simon and Schuster, London

Egan G 1993 Adding value. Josey-Bass, San Francisco

Egan G 1994 Working the shadow side. Josey-Bass, San Francisco

Handy C 1991 Gods of management. Arrow, London

Hellriegel D, Slocum J W, Woodman R W 1998 Organizational behavior, 8th edn. South-Western Publishing, Cincinnati, Ohio

Hersey P, Blanchard K, Johnson D E 1996 Management of organizational behavior: utilizing human resources, 7th edn. Prentice Hall International, London

Janis I L 1972 Groupthink: psychological studies of policy decisions and fiascos. Houghton Mifflin, Boston

Johnson G 1992 Managing strategic change – strategy, culture and actions. Prentice Hall, Englewood Cliffs, NJ

Lewin K 1951 Field theory in social science. Harper and Row, New York

McGregor D C 1960 The human side of enterprise. McGraw Hill, New York

Mullins L J 2002 Management and organisational behaviour. Pitman, London

Senge P M 1990 The fifth discipline. Century Business, London

Tichy N M, Devanna M A 1990 The transformational leader. Wiley, Chichester

Upton T, Brooks B 1995 Managing change in the NHS. Open University Press, Buckingham

The human aspects of organisational change

Application **3:1**
Mark Slattery

Changing roles – same skills, different context!

In this application, Slattery outlines how he needed to change the way he worked when he changed roles from an operational post in an acute hospital to a more strategic environment working on a national strategy. Significantly he points out that the skills themselves are transferable, but it is important to be aware of the influence of the context on both the manager's role and the way people respond to change.

THE NEW ROLE

Over the last 12 months I have changed my role from working in an acute hospital to that of working on a national strategy managed at regional level. This experience has revealed to me a new aspect of the health service, and demonstrated how nurses in strategic roles really can make a difference to how care is delivered at the sharp end.

Twelve months ago I was the clinical manager of the Cardiology, Gastroenterology, Haematology and Oncology Directorates at a 600-bedded hospital in England. My main role was to maintain a service that ensured the delivery of the highest possible standards of care for patients. I also carried out a clinical role by performing oesophageal motility studies and supporting patients with gastroenterological disorders. Supporting and directing the staff that I managed was the most difficult, yet the most rewarding part of the role. It meant working as a team but when difficult decisions had to be made, I was required to make them.

My current role is that of senior project manager. It is very different. In this role, the way I can make a difference to patient care is by influencing others to make changes which then may result in their organisations changing the way patient care is delivered.

In the project management role I work individually, but am supported by my line manager. Previously I worked with (and led) a team with support from a management team. It takes time to adjust to this change in organisational structures and this can result in a feeling of isolation and cause stress. I soon realised that if I was going get through these feelings, I needed to take control of my situation by

Managing and supporting people

reducing my stress and maximising my performance in my new role. I felt that the skills that had allowed me to perform the role of clinical manager (the ability to communicate effectively and to influence, facilitate and support staff through change) could be transferred to a different context and used in my project manager role.

COMMUNICATION

Effective communication is an important tool in achieving effective change. There is more to communication than just talking and listening. You need to believe in what you are trying to communicate; it is then a lot easier to be motivated and to understand what outcomes are aiming at achieving. Knowledge gained by effective communication processes gives the stakeholders more confidence to challenge issues that arise. This gives the information needed to explore the issues before you, as manager, must take on that issue and communicate it to others. (Hendry in Chapter 3 outlines the importance of congruence in achieving effective communication.)

I have found that having the relevant background knowledge has allowed me to answer most of the questions that may be asked as there is time to gather thoughts and think issues through. It is important to be honest and say what you do and don't know, as this will give you credibility with staff. Reflecting back to staff what you think you have heard from them, perhaps by paraphrasing the conversation, is a way to make sure that your intended message has been received.

INFLUENCING OTHERS

The most difficult outcome to achieve within the process of change is to influence others, particularly very senior staff. Not only do you need effective communication skills but you also need to work out how, when and who to influence. This is a process which can only be learnt by doing it in a real-life situation. It is important to maintain transparency and honesty when seeking to influence people, and to develop skills of negotiating in order to achieve best outcomes for the majority of the stakeholders.

The activities in the processes of influencing others require time and ideally some background knowledge of each person. With changing roles and different agendas I found I needed to revisit my influencing skills. I needed to work out who were the people with the authority to make changes. What were their main concerns? What were their main agendas? I was reminded of the key differences between my previous and current roles; the former affected patient care directly while the latter involved working at strategic level, dealing with the political agenda, in order to influence the long-term effects on patient care. I found this more difficult to cope with as it does not have quick results and thus the immediate 'satisfaction' is not present to act as a motivator – it is easy to lose sight of the end product.

FACILITATING AND SUPPORTING OTHERS

The manager 'in the middle' can feel in a 'no win' situation, trying to achieve the expectations of both the staff that they manage and senior management to whom they must answer while trying not to forget about themselves and what they want to achieve personally. This apparent incongruence can cause increased stress levels, which can become intolerable and cause physical symptoms. The use of facilitation techniques is a way around such problems. Encouraging all stakeholder groups to take their share of the responsibility allows for the stress to be shared out.

It is useful – though not always easy – to get all the stakeholders together to try to identify the priorities for each group. Remember that most groups and/or individuals will have their own agenda, and will strive to achieve it, sometimes at the costs of others. Allowing everyone to have their say is a good starting point.

What I had not realised was that some staff's *personal* needs meant so much to them. Once I realised this, I could take it into consideration, although it was important to bear in mind that some of this came from the personal insecurities of the individuals, rather than from the matter under review. To acknowledge and deal with this issue is part of the role of the effective change manager.

CONCLUSION

In my new role I use the same skills as I did in my previous one. I am still pulling different staff groups together so that they work productively with each other and have the same goal of improving patient care, but the goal is further in the future.

As a manager inevitably you have a role in change. To achieve this, you need effective skills of communication, influencing and facilitating. I find that by using these skills I am able to manage my working environment more effectively, and control the stress that I feel while performing my role.

Managing and supporting people

Achieving quality:

moving practice forward through the management of change

In this application, Larsen outlines how a NHS unit intends to treat patients requiring unilateral foot surgery as day cases, rather than as inpatients. Whilst the change is one which is desirable both to patients and the organisation, Larsen points out that it is important to approach the change in a systematic way to achieve the best outcomes. She uses Lewin's model of change to structure the stages in the process. This application is adapted from a project Larsen carried out whilst studying with the Royal College of Nursing to gain a Diploma in Health Service Management.

INTRODUCTION

To achieve effective change, it is important to be clear about the need for it, the triggers which indicate the need for change and who it will affect (i.e. the stakeholders). People are the major factor in any change activity – they influence how effective the outcomes of the change might be. Understanding how the people involved will view and react to the proposal is imperative to the success or failure of the change.

Trigger factors

There is a number of triggers, both internal and external, that inform this change. At a national (political) level are factors that support this change; these factors are central to the Department of Health's document *Shifting the Balance of Power within the NHS* (DoH 2001).

Six Steps to **Effective Management**

An increase in day surgery activity to 75% of all elective surgery is a central feature of *The NHS Plan* (DoH 2000). The ever-increasing pressure of making effective use of available resources questions the appropriateness of current practice. In the locality there is a growing elderly population, which will increase demands on the current service. Advances in medical technology and improved anaesthesia and pain management have contributed to the number of procedures now able to be conducted as day cases.

Internal triggers to the planned change have come from the patients themselves and from some of the clinicians. The increasing pressure for beds and the cancellations of elective surgery have all contributed to the questioning of current practice. Information gained from benchmarking activities in other organisations enabled the Unit to learn from others' successes and mistakes.

Day case versus inpatient surgery

At present in the Unit, patients undergo unilateral foot surgery as inpatients, experiencing an average 3-day stay in hospital. As day case surgery generally is growing in popularity with patients in the UK, an audit was carried out to ascertain the views of patients who had undergone unilateral foot surgery as inpatients. This revealed some interesting findings. The patients reported that they felt the 3-day stay in hospital was very disrupting to their life, suggesting that they would have preferred to have rested at home. A large number of the patients contacted said they would have preferred to be treated as day case patients.

Increasing the amount of day case surgery will reduce waiting lists and waiting times and will lower the costs of health care. Consequently, because of the importance of achieving the maximum health gain from the available resources, purchasers of health care are encouraging provider surgical specialties to undertake a greater proportion of planned caseload as day cases. Two major stakeholders – the patients and the health care purchasers – are thus agreed in principle, and the Unit managers decided to address ways of changing the patterns of admission for this group of patients.

THE CURRENT SITUATION

Patients are admitted to an orthopaedic ward the day prior to their surgery for preoperative assessment. Surgery is performed the next day. On the third day patients are instructed and assessed by a physiotherapist before being discharged. A large number of the multidisciplinary team is involved in the care of these patients. Acute hospital beds are occupied for 3 days.

Managing and supporting people

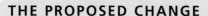

THE PROPOSED CHANGE

It was decided that the Unit would work towards managing patients requiring unilateral foot surgery as day case patients.

Using the selection criteria advocated by the Department of Health (DoH 2002) patients will be assessed in the already existing preoperative assessment clinic as outpatients prior to surgery. This will negate the necessity for patients to be admitted to hospital before surgery. Patients will then attend the day case unit on the day of surgery and will be assessed and instructed by a physiotherapist there. Patients will be discharged on the same day.

CHALLENGES AHEAD – AND WAYS AROUND THEM

- *Cost implications* – The change will require financial, material, manpower and educational input. The aim is to achieve the change in 6 months.
- *Change agent* – To implement change effectively, a change agent must be identified. The role of the change agent is to guide and facilitate the change by skilled analysis of the problem and effective communication.
- *The stakeholders* – A stakeholder analysis will identify those involved, as by encouraging group involvement change is more likely to achieve success. Involving those concerned will help to develop a 'shared vision' and commitment to achieving the change.
- *Commitment planning* – This will address individual stakeholders' level of commitment and where they need to be to implement the change.

CHOOSING A MODEL OF CHANGE – AND APPLYING IT

To consider change, it is useful to determine a model or change strategy that suits the situation. The change proposed must demonstrate it is rational in that it is planned and there are clear reasons for the change. If the change has been initiated from the 'bottom-up', it is described as emergent change.

Change strategies aim to provide a specific pathway of managing change and identification of barriers. Lewin's model of change (1951) is one of the earliest change theories published, and it still has great common sense appeal. Thus it was chosen to act as a framework when planning this change.

Lewin's model describes three steps: unfreezing, moving (changing to a new behaviour) and unfreezing.

Achieving quality: moving practice forward

101

Six Steps to **Effective Management**

Unfreezing

This recognises that a change is required. At the first working party meeting the idea will be discussed in relation to the triggers, and the proposal to move to day case management will be outlined. One of the aims of the meeting will be to identify the resistors and drivers for the proposed change (see Fig. 3.3) using a Force Field analysis tool.

Changing to a new behaviour

Lewin suggests that a process of cognitive redefinition of the problem, i.e. seeking to look at the issues from a new perspective, occurs at this stage. Delegation by the change agent of certain aspects of the change activity, with agreed timescales and milestones, to members of the working party will give them some ownership of the change. Implementation of the proposed change takes place during this period, and the change agent must be prepared to offer support to those involved.

Refreezing

New changes are integrated and stabilised. Reviewing, evaluating and reinforcing the change are important to ensure that things are progressing to plan.

CONCLUSION

The amount of day case surgery undertaken in the UK continues to rise. Indeed the main trigger for this proposed change came from the patients themselves. Continuing to admit otherwise fit patients to carry out unilateral foot surgery will mean to choose a more expensive approach that does not take account of advances in medical and nursing practice. The time spent planning the change, ensuring that staff and patients have relevant information and that processes and systems in the Unit are in place to ensure smooth implementation will have cost implications both in financial terms and in lost opportunity costs. However, once successfully implemented the benefits achieved will be demonstrated in quality of service delivery and in effective resource utilisation.

References

Department of Health 2000 The NHS plan: a plan for investment, a plan for reform. Department of Health, London

Department of Health 2001 Shifting the balance of power within the NHS: securing delivery. Department of Health, London

Department of Health 2002 Day surgery: operational guide. Department of Health, London

Lewin K 1951 Field theory in social science. Harper and Row, New York

Managing and supporting people

Chapter **Four**

Performance management

Debbie Lee

OVERVIEW

In this chapter Lee outlines the rationale, processes and benefits of performance management. She stresses that the process should be seen as joint, i.e. equally shared between employer and employee, and should reap benefits for both parties.

INTRODUCTION

Performance management is a joint process that involves both the supervisor and the employee, to identify common goals, which correlate to the higher goals of the institution. This process results in the establishment of written performance expectations later used as measures for feedback and performance evaluation. (Davis 1995)

As the NHS (National Health Service) and health care generally have become more sophisticated, business systems to measure and evaluate performance have become part of everyday life. This chapter is intended for anyone who manages or is considering the management of performance of others. Whether you are a team leader, an experienced supervisor, a manager or director, this chapter will guide you through the key steps in the performance management process.

But how do you know if you are already involved with the performance management process? The following list will help you identify current responsibilities throughout the process:

- Establishing specific job tasks
- Writing or contributing to the development of job descriptions
- Conducting annual performance reviews
- Being part of a team that develops strategic initiatives that apply to performance standards
- Planning to improve performance
- Establishing or contributing to the development of employee goals.

This chapter will also help you manage performance in order to improve practice and outcomes. By improving understanding and learning to work collaboratively with employees and colleagues you will be able to:

- identify an employee's core job description in line with the organisation's mission
- identify key steps that are appropriate to support an individual in meeting personal goals and the goals of the organisation
- develop realistic and appropriate performance standards
- give and receive effective feedback about performance
- write and undertake constructive performance reviews
- plan education and development opportunities that will enable individuals to deliver performance standards
- work with individuals and teams to improve current performance.

As part of developing understanding in the field of performance management, look for information within your own organisation. By doing this you will discover a wealth of useful processes that will help you establish an effective and appropriate performance management framework. Things to consider include:

- obtaining copies of personnel policies and procedures
- making contact with your personnel department (most units will have a link person who will be only too happy to assist you)
- speaking to a professional officer or union representative who will have the latest information on national policies and agendas

Managing and supporting people

- enrolling in training and educational programmes that focus on performance management
- looking at the internet for useful resources such as http://www.doh.gov.uk/hrstrategy/index.htm and http://www.doh.gov.uk.

NHS POLICY

Managing the performance of staff so that we can ensure effective and efficient delivery of services has not become a top priority by accident. *The NHS Plan* (DoH 2000a) has identified the importance of having the right calibre of staff in the right place at the right time, in order to deliver a modernised health service that the public deserve and have grown to expect. If you can access your bank from home 24 hours a day every day of the year then why can't you do the same with health care? Equally, staff working in health care have for far too long worked under difficult circumstances with little reward to show for their efforts. Recruitment and more importantly retaining staff has dominated all strategic plans and policies. By investing in its staff and improving working lives it is envisaged that this will contribute significantly to the problem, thus ensuring that the health service becomes a place where we are all proud to work, and aid in the recruitment and retention of the most valuable resource – staff.

The government's modernisation strategy is comprised of three strands: quality improvement, information and staff. Back in early 2000 national priorities guidance was issued to all NHS providers. The guidance laid out a human resources performance framework (DoH 2000b) that was aimed at all staff working in the NHS in liaison with social services at a local level. Within the framework three performance objectives were identified:

- Improving working lives
- Working together
- Developing the workforce.

The then regional offices had the overall responsibility for ensuring delivery of the national targets.

Improving working lives

Making the NHS an attractive place to work and being able to encourage a new generation to make health care its career became a

Performance management

> **Box 4.1** The Improving Working Lives standard
>
> An employer committed to the IWL standard:
> - recognises that modern health services require modern employment services of working patterns
> - understands that staff work best for patients when they can strike a health balance between work and other aspects of their life outside work
> - accepts joint responsibility with staff to develop a range of working arrangements that balance the needs of the patients and the services with the needs of staff
> - values and supports staff according to the contribution they make to patient care and meeting the needs of the service
> - provides personal and professional development and training opportunities that are accessible and open to all staff
> - has a range of policies and practices that enable staff to manage a healthy balance between work and their outside commitments.

top priority in order to deliver modernised services. To achieve this the *Improving Working Lives* (IWL) campaign was launched in 1999 (DoH 1999a). Clear standards were laid out to develop an environment that supports staff and protects their welfare. Staff complained of a long hours culture and a lack of balance between work and home life. Task forces were established regionally to promote the strategy and support organisations with implementation with an expectation that by April 2003 all NHS employers would meet IWL standards.

The IWL standard is outlined in Box 4.1.

Working together

Working Together: Securing a Quality Workforce was launched in 1998 (DoH 1998) and was another significant stake in the ground to improve standards of human resource management. Specifically, planning targets stated that:

- all primary care trusts are to develop plans for implementing the human resource standards as set out in the *Human Resource Guidance and Requirements for Primary Care Trusts* (issued in December 1999, DoH 1999b)
- employers have a set deadline for all health professional staff to have training and development plans linked to an agreed system of appraisal
- employers must have met the criteria to use the Employment Service Symbol

- Greater scope to create new kinds of jobs, with the objectives of bringing about more patient-centred care and more motivated NHS staff
- A fairer pay system based on structured analysis
- Harmonised conditions of service for NHS staff
- A more transparent reward system for staff who work outside the more traditional working hours
- Improved links between career and pay progression.

To support personal development a new *NHS Knowledge and Skills Framework* is being developed. This will support the process of annual performance management reviews and become the mechanism for agreeing your personal development plan. Elements being made available include:

- Everyone will be expected to develop their skills and the knowledge needed to further improve performance or service delivery
- The NHS Knowledge and Skills Framework will help to identify the knowledge and skills needed for each post
- Each individual will have a development review meeting with their manager each year to agree development for the next year
- Each individual will agree a personal development plan which will describe how learning will be supported each year (see Application 4:2)
- Successful development will allow individuals to progress up the pay points until they reach the top of their band.

The system will provide for better links to be made for all NHS staff between education, development and career planning, and pay progression. Each member of staff will have a personal development plan, and for each part of that plan clear support mechanisms will be identified. Their plan will help individuals to build for the future, ensuring that they are obtaining the right skills and knowledge, not only for their current job but also those that will apply to their future career. The aims are that all staff should:

- have clear, consistent development objectives
- be helped to develop in such a way that they can apply the knowledge and skills to their level of responsibility
- be helped to identify and develop knowledge and skills that will support their career progression.

Basic pay will be decided through job evaluation and a new NHS job evaluation scheme will be used to cover all new posts. The correct pay band will be determined only after a detailed assessment has taken place. The roll out of the *Agenda for Change* (DoH 2003) has already led to many posts being evaluated nationally; however, posts that are more unusual will be evaluated at a local level.

STRATEGIC PLAN

The development of the concept of performance management as a new human resource management model has reflected a change in the management style in the NHS from a 'top-down, command and control' approach to that of a more facilitative 'people friendly' leader. This change has been recognised and supported by central government, and more importantly values employees and their level of performance in delivering the long-term goals of the health service.

Employees' goals originate from their work departments which must support the organisation's overall missions and goals. A performance management framework provides the employer and employee with a systematic process to discuss the development of goals and to create jointly a plan that will enable the successful delivery of those goals. A development plan should support this process, which will enable the employee to grow professionally and contribute effectively to the organisational goals.

The rapidly changing environment means that both employer and employee need to be flexible and adaptive in order to solve problems effectively. Employers need to be able to respond to changes, work creatively and communicate effectively to many diverse groups. To complement this, an employee needs to take responsibility for personal development, be able to learn how to keep apace of change and anticipate the future challenges within the workplace.

Where to begin

A starting place for performance management and developing your strategic plan is writing a job description. This is an important process of analysing data and collecting key facts about a job. When a vacancy is identified a job description is produced before advertising the job. This process must fit cohesively with the organisation's mission and goals. Once the employee has been appointed, the job description becomes the initial basis for job delivery, outlining the outcomes to be achieved. This should be reviewed on a planned basis with the line manager to measure progress of delivery of objectives. A job description should specify:

- the specific job functions and outcomes
- elements of the role that are desirable and essential
- an indication of the percentage of time allocated to each function
- the skills knowledge and abilities (or level of competency required) to perform the job
- the academic level and physical ability required to do the job
- any special conditions of service
- the level of supervision that will be exercised.

As part of the employee's induction process, usually during the first few days of starting a new job, the manager should guide the employee through the job description, ensuring there is clarity of understanding. A record should then be made that this process has been undertaken, outlining the outcomes agreed.

Supporting this process is a strategic plan, which will be an integral part of the overall organisational plan. The plan is built on the foundation of the mission statement, with clearly identifiable goals. The mission statement should identify why the organisation exists, with personal goals identified to support the delivery of the mission. The strategic plan sets out specific steps that must be taken to achieve the agreed results. The development of a strategic plan is a dynamic process, which is usually revisited on an annual basis.

Individual employees should be given the opportunity to contribute to the strategic plan, ensuring that priorities for action are identified and ownership of delivery is attained. Within the strategic plan goals are identified, strategies and initiatives are outlined and responsibilities (with completion dates) are made explicit.

As a performance manager, you should be able to analyse essential data and consider annual goals for each employee. Each employee will need clarity of role and level of responsibility; standards or levels of competence should be set for work performance. Employees will need feedback on their performance. This varies from organisation to organisation but most practice supports an annual review, with regular updates in between. As part of the strategic plan, resources need to be made available to support education, training and development that can be delivered flexibly to meet the needs of the individual and the organisation, thus contributing to quality service delivery.

STANDARDS OF PERFORMANCE

A standard of performance is a written statement explicitly outlining how a job should be performed. Standards can be written collaboratively between employers and employees and should be used as part of annual reviews and updates on service delivery.

The performance standard is a useful benchmark that can be used as a learning tool to evaluate outcomes. It is a useful tool that will provide information on whether an individual is meeting or exceeding the role expectations. A job description is there to describe the essential functions of a job. The performance standard identifies to what level a function should be delivered. Most managers have criteria that they use to evaluate performance, ensuring that they measure 'like for like'. For some organisations this becomes the mechanism to rate employees for their level of pay increase, rewarding individuals for their annual achievements.

The development of performance standards can be approached in two ways:

- a *directive approach*, where the performance manager alone writes the standards (this will still need consultation with employee relations representatives and employees affected by the standards).
- a *collaborative approach*, where employers work in partnership with employees to develop performance standards.

The final responsibility lies with the performance manager who decides on the appropriateness of standards in relation to the organisation's mission and goals. When writing standards consider learning from others. Why reinvent the wheel? If a similar unit has already undertaken this process, the results may provide a useful foundation from which to start. Your human resource department will guide you on frameworks and structures, ensuring that there is equality and equity demonstrated throughout the whole organisation.

When the standards are in draft format, consultation with all appropriate staff is essential. Staff need to be made aware of the content of the standard and fully understand the implications. Effective communication at this stage is vital. Encourage comments and questioning and allow enough time for all staff to get involved. Remember that those on shift work, particularly night duty, will still want an opportunity to comment, so plan for this.

When writing performance standards a good starting point is to obtain copies of:

- current job descriptions
- the organisation's business plan including mission statements and goals
- all current forms used to appraise staff
- any previous standards used
- standards from other units
- relevant organisational policies
- relevant local and national policies.

For effective communication make sure that you write everything in plain English, with a focus on the minimum competencies and outcomes that will be measured. The standards should be for the job, not for the specific person undertaking the job. Remember to make the standards reasonable and appropriate. The standard should describe your expectations and have a built-in mechanism for acceptability of errors. This needs serious consideration in terms of clinical risk management, as for some standards it will be acceptable to allow for a margin of error whereas for others relating to clinical practice, it may not. The following pointers are useful to consider when writing standards:

- Relate the standards to specific job requirements
- Include a reporting system that can measure relevant quantitative data
- For performance standards that concentrate on qualitative aspects of a job ensure you describe clearly the specific characteristics required that can be verified
- Include links to organisational objectives in order to ensure that the corporate agenda is achieved.

Once you have written the standards ask yourself the following questions:

- Are the standards realistic and consistent across the organisation?
- Are the standards specific, so that the employee is clear about all the outcomes to be achieved?
- Are the standards based on data that can be measured (e.g. in terms of cost, time, quality and quantity)?
- Are the standards consistent with the goals of the organisation and do they fall in line with the mission statement?
- Will the standards be challenging? (We all need motivating in our work and need something to strive towards.)

Performance management

- Are the standards clear and unambiguous; can the employees understand them?
- Are the standards dynamic, incorporating the flexibility to adapt to our ever changing environment?
- Have good communication networks been established when producing these standards? For example you may wish to consult:
  —Management
  —Human resource links
  —Training and education
  —Nursing services
  —Professions allied to medicine
  —Medical profession
  —Support services
  —Voluntary sector
  —Services users.

All staff groups are interrelated; they cannot function in isolation if they are to deliver services effectively.

Observation and feedback

The process of observing staff performance and providing feedback should take place as part of a continuous process. A routine should be established for formal feedback and built into the performance management process. All feedback given should be based on facts that have been obtained from observed behaviours, actions taken, statements made and results achieved. Using your time effectively will help an employee to attain a good standard of performance. By supporting and guiding an employee, new skills will be learnt and planned outcomes achieved. Providing feedback very often reinforces the aspects of the job that has to be delivered and will instil confidence in individuals who may be struggling over the delivery of complex tasks. When observing staff make sure you record specific facts such as time, date, specific events and the employee's approach in delivering objectives. This will aid individuals to develop their skills knowledge and abilities and enable them to develop within a changing and complex environment.

There will be times when you will not be present to observe performance. Careful consideration needs to be given to your systems and processes so that employees are assessed effectively.

Employees will need to understand the processes used and feel confident that they are being assessed fairly and openly. When assessing performance that has occurred in your absence, you may wish to consider the following aspects:

- Evaluate the outcomes of the employees' work
- Have routine planned meetings with your staff; this will be an opportunity to discuss performance and reduce anxieties on delivery of objectives
- Routinely discuss employees' standards of performance with them; feedback should not be a shock, it should be given via a continual process of development
- Encourage employees to provide written updates on progress; this will help you map out developments in line with the corporate agendas
- Obtain feedback from those using the service; it is because of them that we are all here in the first place
- Obtain feedback from employees and peers, ensuring that there is common understanding of roles and responsibilities
- Undertake routine spot checks of employees in their workplace; this will give you valuable information on their day-to-day delivery of work
- Use phone calls and emails to obtain feedback from employees; sometimes just by asking how an individual is can open up some important issues.

Most of us give behavioural feedback; this will be a clear statement on observed behaviour. Consider the following when you are using this type of feedback:

- Try to base your feedback on verified data that relate to the observed behaviour (e.g. date, time, place)
- Give the employee an opportunity to describe observed behaviour and the rationale for it before you give your feedback. There may be a valid reason for an individual's behaviour which will influence your thinking and any action to be taken
- Always explain the impact of the employee's behaviour on others and on the organisation. This will help the employee relate to the overall relevance of actions and identify what actions are important
- Ensure the location you choose to give feedback respects the individual's need for privacy and avoids annoying interruptions that may break the flow of conversation.

Performance management

Performance appraisal

A performance appraisal is a process of assessing the development of an employee and making a summary of it. The process should be set up so that feedback can be two-way (employer–employee), ensuring that the employee feels relaxed enough to be able to share how they think they have done since their last appraisal and how they feel they were supported. The employer needs to be as objective as possible in this process, and should have planned ahead by obtaining evidence to give feedback on performance. Preparation is key in the success of the performance appraisal.

The following steps may help you get yourself ready:

1. Before the meeting takes place with the employee make sure you have a copy of, and have read, the job description and the previous performance review records
2. Review your own observations and those you have obtained from relevant others
3. Don't forget to include feedback from members of the employee's team and those to whom you are delivering a service
4. If the employee reports to more than one manager, make sure that you have agreed with the other manager(s) the process and content of feedback
5. If there is a performance problem, make sure that you are aware of who knows about it; this can be a very sensitive part of the process and confidentiality will need to be carefully considered
6. Make sure the employee has plenty of notice of when the performance review will take place and how long it will take; this will give individuals time to reflect and prepare for the meeting
7. Wherever possible, try to see the employee before the performance review; this will ensure that there is clarity of the process for the employee before the review meeting actually takes place
8. At the meeting ensure that you have an appropriate environment to undertake the performance review
9. Always explain the process to the employee as an introduction to the performance review
10. Follow the performance review model used in your organisation to ensure fairness and consistency
11. Always allow plenty of time for discussion and questioning

12. Conclude the meeting so that both the employer and employee have clarity on what has been discussed and what has been agreed; this will need to be written down for future reference

13. Schedule the next performance review meeting before the session concludes.

When writing up the performance appraisal ensure that each part of the document is completed and make sure that you consider the following:

- How does the employee's performance compare with the performance standards of the job?
- How did you confirm the level of performance achieved by the employee?
- What are the consequences of the level of performance achieved?

When you are delivering your performance review, remember that this is a formal process. However well you know an individual, never be tempted to cut corners. It is good practice to ask the employee, prior to the appraisal, to undertake a self-assessment to be shared during the process. This will help you identify how self-aware an individual is and to provide an opportunity to bring new information to the meeting.

The objectives of the discussion should include:

- a review of the job description and how much effort the employee has made to deliver the job description
- identification of strengths and areas for improvement
- a review of the outcomes of last year's performance appraisal and a sharing of accomplishments
- sharing corporate strategy, ensuring that the employee is clear where and how they fit into that strategy
- discussing areas of agreement and difference:

You should both sign a copy of the final performance appraisal. A copy is given to the employee. The whole process should be about getting the best out of individuals and be a mechanism for efficient and effective communication. The overall objective is to enable employees to do an effective job, and to plan for the future in a way that is constructive and motivational for both parties.

Performance development

An important component of the performance management process is the production of a personal development plan. This will provide

Performance management

another opportunity for collaborative working, developing skill, knowledge and abilities with the support from relevant others. There can be a number of reasons why you choose to instigate a performance development plan and these may be:

- as part of the regular performance review process
- a demonstrated need of an area for improvement following an incident
- when an employee requests a particular development opportunity
- as part of the wider corporate agenda.

The development plan should be a balance between the needs of the individual and the needs of the organisation. When planning the delivery of the development plan use a flexible approach that meets the needs of the employee and the needs of the service. Some methods to consider include:

- online and distance learning packages
- attending programmes provided by higher education
- on the job training
- attending conferences, meetings or committees
- coaching and mentoring
- shadowing
- participating or leading a project
- writing articles or books
- participating in or being a member of professional organisations
- utilising technology such as teleconferencing, or the internet.

CONCLUSION

Performance management processes should demonstrate a structured approach that will support you in having the right people, in the right place, at the right time. It will provide the employer with useful data on outcomes and a mechanism that will support benchmarking of services. Overall it will support the growth of individuals and services, build on and improve the motivation of the team, and facilitate commitment and loyalty to the organisation. The performance management process begins with analysis of the job under review; this is in line with the organisation's mission and goals. It sets the minimum standards required to deliver the job and directs individuals to strive for better results. National policy will continue to see this as a vital step to modernise the NHS and will remain on all our agendas for some time into the future.

Discussion questions

- What are the key objectives of performance review?
- What must you consider when preparing a job description and/or a person specification?
- How would you go about ensuring that the elements within an individual review are relevant to the organisation?
- How can the process of performance review contribute to the personal development of individuals?
- What sources of information might a manager use when preparing to carry out a performance review?

References

Davis R 1995 Choosing performance management: a holistic approach. CUPA Journal (USA) Summer

Department of Health 1998 Working together: securing a quality workforce. Department of Health, London

Department of Health 1999a Improving working lives. Department of Health, London

Department of Health 1999b Human resource guidance and requirements for primary care trusts. Department of Health, London

Department of Health 2000a The NHS plan: a plan for investment, a plan for reform. Department of Health, London

Department of Health 2000b Human resources performance framework. Department of Health, London

Department of Health 2003 Agenda for change, the new NHS pay system – an overview. Department of Health, London

Performance management

Application **4:1**

E Nichols

Performance management applied:

managing staff sickness

In this application, Nichols outlines a very real issue and how the introduction of processes of performance management can contribute to improving services. She also emphasises a very important point: performance management should not be seen as a punitive activity, but as a developmental one, from which all participants should benefit.

INTRODUCTION

During my time as clinical manager of a large acute directorate covering three sites, a method of performance management evolved in response to external scrutiny of practice and to address questions asked by the Trust management team about efficiency and adherence to trust policies and procedures. Statistics comparing directorates were available to the Trust on several issues. The example of sickness absence illustrates how this issue might be addressed via the process of performance management across a unit of any size.

HISTORY OF THE ISSUE

Staff absences were consistently high in the directorate when compared to others. Over almost a year the absence figures for the directorate were fairly constant for both long- and short-term sickness. The directorate was asked to explain the figures as it was perceived to be inefficient. A very detailed analysis of the workforce in the directorate took place to try to identify the problem and establish a baseline. The main conclusions were:

● In medicine there is a lower qualified staff ratio per bed than in other areas

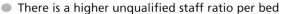 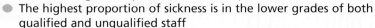

- There is a higher unqualified staff ratio per bed
- The highest proportion of sickness is in the lower grades of both qualified and unqualified staff
- The directorate had a significantly higher number of staff over the age of 50 than any other directorate
- Ward managers were not strictly following the 'management of absence' policy, as they saw it as not having 'teeth' and thus felt powerless to carry out any action on this aspect of their job.

When the analysis was complete there was no quick fix that could be applied. Action had to be taken due to the cost pressure and constant overspend that staff sickness was creating, as it was at least 4% above the funding built into the ward budgets. The key to addressing the issue was seen as getting the ward managers to own the problem, and to support and empower them through advice in dealing with staff absences. Staff also had to be able to see that the ward managers did monitor individuals and take action. It was intended that eventually an attitude shift could be effected in all grades of staff that would lead to reducing absences and the reliance on bank and agency staff.

FIRST APPROACH VIA PERFORMANCE MANAGEMENT

Following debate about sickness and other issues in the directorate, a strategy was agreed to launch the issues with the ward managers, encourage discussion, agree an action plan and monitor its effectiveness. A 'time out day' was held for the ward managers facilitated by an external person. The facilitator was briefed in advance of the issues that would be raised and that needed to be tackled. An action plan and the monitoring mechanism were agreed and implemented. The ward managers were expected to know the relevant policies within which they were to operate.

It was agreed that instead of the absence figures being provided to the ward managers, the ward managers would use part of the local sisters' meeting to report formally on their individual areas. At this meeting they could discuss confidentially particular problems and solutions in a supportive manner among their peers. The directorate general manager was also present, participating fully and often giving advice. The directorate personnel advisor attended as requested. The minutes of the meeting summarised issues and action plans for the ward areas.

After about 18 months this approach did not achieve significant results. Staff sickness did reduce by about 1% but continued to be high and fluctuate widely. The management of absence policy was still seen not to assist the ward manager in managing.

Performance management applied: managing staff sickness

SECOND APPROACH VIA PERFORMANCE MANAGEMENT

Sickness levels across nursing staff in the Trust continued to be higher than those of any other grade of staff and were examined as a result. This led to a review of the management of absence policy. This provided the platform to re-launch the management of sickness for all staff employed in the Trust. Before launching the new policy the directorate considered how this would be done, who should be involved and what the outcomes from the policy and its implementation should be.

Communication

Communication of the new absence policy was initially done by paper circulation to all departmental/ward managers. The clinical manager, general manager and personnel advisor then reinforced this through the local ward manager's meetings for the nursing staff. A full mandatory training day on the topic was then held for all ward managers along with the clinical and other managerial staff. This ensured that everyone:

- had the same interpretation of the policy
- had received the same training
- had an opportunity to work through scenarios
- understood that there was definite action that could be taken with individuals where a problem was identified.

Implementation

The policy now had to be implemented by the ward managers in their areas. Each ward manager took the policy back and briefed their staff on the process that would be followed for reporting and managing absences. The policy was made available to all staff.

Monitoring

Monthly review meetings were established between the clinical manager, site senior nurse and the individual ward managers to review sickness and financial matters. A standing agenda was agreed for these meetings and notes kept. The overall level of sickness was considered and areas of low levels were examined to see what lessons could be passed on to others. In wards that had a high incidence of sickness the individual staff were considered at the meeting. An action plan to manage them was agreed at the meeting and implemented before the next one. The action agreed was recorded and reviewed at the next meeting. This format ensured

Managing and supporting people

continuity of application of the policy and process in a timely manner as well as guidance and support in the application of the process. A personnel advisor and the Occupational Health Department supported the ward managers in their action. The ward managers owned the process, action and the results that they achieved. As the pattern of the meetings became established, and the skills of the ward managers developed, it was no longer necessary for the clinical manager to attend each meeting.

The results achieved varied from month to month and continued to demonstrate a sustained reduction in the average sickness absence rate (Table 4.1.1). This approach helped to reduce the financial pressure due to temporary staffing costs to cover unexpected absences.

PERFORMANCE MANAGEMENT DEVELOPMENT

Since this management approach was established within the clinical directorate, a significant reorganisation and expansion of services has taken place following the merger of two Trusts. This management approach was further developed and adopted to manage resources more widely as well as aspects of staff development, personnel issues and clinical governance. A standard reporting system was developed and implemented to support this process and set a standing agenda to match the priorities of the Trust and directorate.

Management of staff absences continues to be a priority in the new Trust. During the first year of the merged Trust, staff absences rose significantly and within the directorate reached 6.8%. Within 1 year of the application of the new performance framework the level of absences was consistently at least 1% lower than in the previous year and the ward managers had become proactive and knowledgeable in implementing plans to manage individual members of their teams.

Table 4.1.1 Sickness absence rates prior to and following performance management (reproduced with kind permission of North Bristol NHS Trust)

	Prior to action (%)	Rates achieved after first approach (%)	Rates achieved after second approach (%)
Hospital 1	6.7	5.5	2.5
Hospital 2	8.1	6.9	5.8
Hospital 3	7.3	9.0	5.0

CONCLUSION

Performance management is the term being used at present to describe the management of Trusts, units or individuals based on their success against targets or objectives set for them. This is not a new concept and has previously been implicit, for example, through mechanisms such as the appraisal system for staff, benchmarking of aspects of an organisation or the compilation of reports across an organisation comparing units and their performance against contracts.

Performance management is a tool that is increasingly being introduced into many aspects of the health service as well as into individuals' job content. Performance management should not be used in isolation or it can be misconstrued as negative and seen only as a big stick. If used correctly as part of an overall approach to managing, then performance management can increase the effectiveness of a unit manager as well as ensuring good regular communication between themselves and the key personnel in the unit. Performance management will not work if those who are being measured are not sufficiently educated/trained or informed about the issues being managed and the relevant policies, procedures, standards and frameworks, etc.

Key aspects that must be present in performance management are outlined in Box 4.1.1.

Box 4.1.1 Key aspects of performance management

- Set objectives for the unit and inform key personnel about how they can contribute to the delivery of these
- Establish constructive, regular, two-way communication between the unit manager and their staff in an ever-changing climate
- Ensure effective delegation of appropriate work or action
- Establish a monitoring system of delegated action
- Provide support and mentoring for key individuals
- Provide a method of managing poor performers
- Provide a regular structure to give encouragement and praise to those who are performing
- Establish the baseline education/training requirements of key staff to fulfil their management role
- Ensure correct interpretation, application and adherence to policies within an organisation
- Stimulate revision or the development of new policies to respond to changing culture, practice or law.

Making personal development plans work for you

In this application Hyde suggests that taking charge of your own personal development is easier than you might think, and that by keeping an ongoing plan, you will be ready to make the most of every opportunity.

INTRODUCTION

In Chapter Four Lee points out the importance of active personal development processes which can also contribute to appraisal activities within the overall process of performance management. Chapter Six includes reference to the self-development model devised by Hyde & Wright (1997) which takes a strategic approach to self-development. Individual personal development plans (PDPs) help you to focus on particular areas of your life, and to craft an ongoing action plan to achieve your goals. Chapter Seven encourages you to do this within a 'whole self' context to achieve balance and wellbeing.

In the broadest sense, we all have the opportunity to develop personally from anything we do in either our personal or professional life. This development activity is congruent with the framework of lifelong learning and should be grounded in each of us, as individuals, rather than being dependent wholly on any one organisation.

PLANNING A PDP

Personal development plans should be flexible, responsive to change, and above all easy to maintain. They should not be produced in isolation from your other professional or personal activity, and should allow you to keep your options open!

The fast changing context of health care produces challenges for PDP preparation. Today a 3–5 year time window is definitely long term in planning scales – whereas 20 years ago, long-term personal planning was more likely to address a time window of 10 years.

Think for a moment what you were doing this time last year – how much has that changed – or remained relatively constant? And why?

Personal development planning can sometimes result in making a conscious and informed choice to do nothing – despite the implicit assumption that one must always be doing something. Doing nothing in the context of active PDP activity can be likened to a farmer laying a field fallow. Whilst apparently nothing is growing (i.e. developing) in reality a lot is going on! Laying fallow (in agricultural terms) is a time of regeneration, of consolidation and of gathering strength. There are times in personal and professional life when this is appropriate too.

The 'rule of three'

When planning personal development, it is useful to bear in mind the 'rule of three'. Most people can divide their activities and responsibilities into three sections: family/friends, professional and personal/individual. Most people can cope with changes in two out of the three, but if there is significant change happening (even if it is welcome change) in all three, life becomes a bit hectic. Thus a period of fallow in one corner of life can be helpful to counteract change in other parts. This can only be a general model as there are so many variables in relation to people and their responsibilities. Nevertheless it makes the point that everything and every facet of life has the potential to become a development opportunity – even if it is not always what one might think!

Choosing the route to self-development

A PDP is a self-devised plan which maps out the route an individual chooses to take to achieve personal and professional goals. A PDP serves as a basis for self-development activity, a basis for discussion at appraisal meetings, and a mechanism to identify strengths, preferences and development needs which can then inform future activity. In short, it allows you to take stock of your life. It is also an important tool for establishing areas of work, lifestyle, etc. that definitely do not appeal – for it is as important to know what you *do not* want as to know what you do want. This might relate to job content, location or context. For example, some people thrive on working with large groups of people, whilst others prefer to work alone, or in a small group.

STARTING A PDP

To start your PDP ask yourself three questions:

1. Where am I now?
2. What do I want to be doing in 1 year; 3 years; 5 years?
3. What do I need to do to achieve this?

1. Where am I now – and what have I achieved to get here?

You might like to consider some of the following points:

- Life experiences plus skills gained in work and non-work environments
- Past employment history, role, responsibilities, but most importantly, what has been gained from the experiences
- Academic and/or vocational courses: what was gained besides the qualification?
- What am I very good at, what do I know I need to develop, and what do I *not* want to do?

To help you do this, try to do the following exercise:

- Write down five things, in order of preference, that are important to you in (a) your personal life, and (b) your job.

This list will help you focus on what is important to you.

2. What do I want to be doing in 1 year; 3 years; 5 years?

Aim high! This means that you should be true to yourself about what you *want* to be doing, but it should not be qualified with 'But I can't because of ...'. You must first focus on your goal, and then think laterally. Remember what Sherlock Holmes said: 'Whenever you have eliminated the impossible, whatever remains, however improbable, is the truth'. The thrust of this dictat is that one should consider every option and discard nothing initially, however improbable it may seem!

3. What do I need to do to achieve this?

Once you have identified your aims/goals, consider what you need to do to achieve them, and set yourself broad timeframes within which to work. You may find it useful to make notes within a simple framework such as the one suggested in Figure 4.2.1. Some people find that it is helpful to have a discussion with a trusted friend, colleague or mentor to help get past the problem of 'not seeing the wood for the trees'. Developing an awareness of self and our

Making personal development plans work for you

127

Aim/goal (Personal or professional)	Details of the aim/goal broken down into small chunks	When do I want it to happen?	How I am going to progress it?
Developmental and/or training need (Remember this may be informal, e.g. shadowing, or more formal, e.g. attendance on a course)	Details of the need	When does it have to start?	How am I going to meet the need?
Resources required (Material and/or people)	What resources?	When will I need to have them?	How will I get them?
Financial implications (Outlay and/or lost opportunity costs)	Are there any?	If so, when will they bite?	How can I prepare for these?

Date:

Review date: *(usually 6 months)*

developmental needs is something that improves with practice. The effort put into it pays dividends both professionally and personally. Good luck!

Reference

Hyde J, Wright A 1997 Self development. Nursing Management 4(3): 10–11

Chapter **Five**

Leadership and management

Michael J Cook

- Leadership within the NHS
- Leadership, management, administration
- Contingency theory
- Unexpected events
- Mentorship
- Preceptorship
- Clinical supervision
- Stress

OVERVIEW

In this chapter Cook focuses on two issues in relation to the debate on leadership and management. Firstly the difference between administration, management and leadership and secondly the importance of mentorship, preceptorship and clinical supervision for supporting staff. He provides a theoretical overview of leadership and management and comments on the importance of achieving a balance between each of these aspects in daily work.

INTRODUCTION

There is no doubt that the National Health Service (NHS) is an environment of constant turmoil, partially due to the lack of agreement as to the strategic priorities (Baggott 1998, Warner et al 1998). This turmoil has placed significant pressure on staff working in the NHS (Burkitt et al 2000). This is a reflection of a world which is changing from an industrial age of the 20th century to the quantum age of the 21st century. The quantum age is one where technological changes are generating incrementally faster changes to living. The impact of these changes is difficult to predict and very difficult to control (Wheatley 1994, Capra 1997). For these reasons health care staff have to learn to lead and manage in this turbulent environment.

Conventional bureaucratic hierarchies, top-down leadership and autocratic management will not be effective in meeting the significant challenges being experienced by staff in health care. Leaders and managers will have to generate speedy responses, learn to work in flatter, less hierarchical organisations, where roles and jobs are more flexible, with higher and broader skill levels, and greater expectations of close involvement in decision making from both employer and employee (Porter-O'Grady 1994, Norman 1995).

These developments require the health service to change, and this is leading to a review of the way that people are led and managed. Joiner (1994) and Dahlgaard et al (1997) identify that effective leadership is a major determinant in the success of organisations. Bolman & Deal (1991, p. 403) state that it is usual for 'leadership to be offered as a solution for most of the problems of organisations everywhere'. And so it is in nursing that effective nursing leadership is cited as a major factor that will improve patient care (Cunningham & Whitby 1997, Cook 1999, Allen 2000).

MANAGEMENT AND LEADERSHIP IN THE NHS

Within the NHS emphasis has been placed on both management and leadership. Management, and in particular the importance of employing modern management skills, was emphasised in the 1980s with the publication of the Griffiths Report (DHSS 1983). This ethos was further reinforced during the Conservative government of the 80s and the 90s with the creation of an internal market for the NHS. More recently, the call for leadership has been offered as *the* resolution.

Yet, even with this emphasis on management and leadership within the NHS, signs of management and leadership failure exist. Deming (1986) actually argues that managers create 85–90% of organisational problems. One report indicates that high levels of psychological disturbance, ranging from emotional exhaustion to suicide, exist in 29–49% of nurses and that much of this ill health is associated with aspects of work (Williams et al 1998). Similar figures are reported in the same publication for medical staff and therapists. Noting this trend of increased ill health amongst health care workers, senior staff in the NHS have recognised a need for change and called for the introduction of a 'servant leader' ethos amongst those who serve the NHS, placing emphasis on leadership to the detriment of effective management (Jarrold 1998).

A swing from management to leadership seems to have occurred, but to bring about sustained change within the NHS requires a balance of inspirational leadership and effective management, coupled with strong administration.

The call for leadership within the National Health Service

Good leadership is required to achieve good quality care (Booth 1995, Hulatt 1995, Rowden 1995, Maggs 1996, Sams 1996, Benton 1997, Connolly 1997, Smith 1997, Salvage 1999, Allen 2000). This emphasis on leadership for all NHS clinical services has been emphasised in several policy documents: *The New NHS: Modern, Dependable* (DoH 1997), *A First Class Service: Quality in the New NHS* (DoH 1998). The nursing, midwifery and health visiting strategy *Making a Difference* (DoH 1999) contained a whole section devoted to strengthening leadership, in which it was stated 'the government's modernisation programme means that more nurses ... need better leadership skills'. None of the above documents, however, defines nursing leadership, and many seem to be interpreting effective leadership as the all-controlling 'super-manager'. It is therefore important to define what each of these terms mean. So what do the terms management and leadership mean?

Definition of management

Management definitions tend to encapsulate the view that the role of the manager is to achieve the objectives of the organisation through the resources available, resources referring to people and tangible artefacts, such as materials. It is useful to note that the definition does not indicate that the manager is involved in setting the objectives of the organisation.

Definition of leadership

Definitions of leadership abound from the great person theory, to the skills attributes stance to the now almost universally accepted

Leadership and management

contingency view of leadership. The following captures in a very brief but meaningful way the differences between leadership and management. In addition a third role, administration, is introduced as a third leg to the stool of organisational efficiency and effectiveness.

Leadership, management, administration

> Leadership is about path making, doing right things. Management is about path following, doing things right. Administration is about path tidying, doing things. (West-Burnham 1998).

People working in organisations have aspects of each of these roles in their day-to-day work. People who are more successful seem to be able to achieve the right balance of each role and know what and when to delegate aspects of the role to others. Delegation includes delegation to peers, those one supervises and one's own supervisor.

Figure 5.1 shows the interrelationship between each of the three roles and how each impacts on the other. Figure 5.2 shows how at

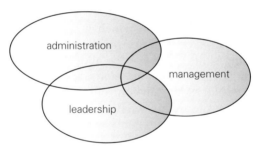

Figure 5.1 Interrelationships between leadership, management and administration

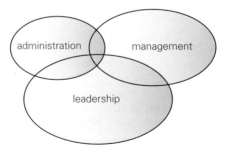

Figure 5.2 Interrelationship change throughout the day

various points even within the same day, it is possible for people to have a greater emphasis on any of the three areas of activity. It is a useful exercise to identify the predominant aspect of one's own role and to ask if the balance is appropriate. After identifying the range of activities and allocated each to an area of administration, leadership or management, the next useful step is to ask why is one involved in a particular task. Is this habit or convenience? Is best use being made of the time and resources available?

STYLES OF MANAGEMENT AND LEADERSHIP

Styles of management and leadership have been written about extensively and repetition is not useful in this short chapter. However, what is becoming apparent is that with respect to questions on the correct management or leadership style then the answer from most writers is 'it depends'. This is referred to as 'contingency theory' and is the belief that to achieve change (the essential element of any management or leadership position) effective leaders do whatever the circumstances require. The theory seems to say that if the world changes then the style of leadership must change. Few writers, researchers and thinkers seem to question this wisdom. Yet an important element of effective leadership is trust and integrity and this means respecting co-workers as equals. Whilst many definitions exist with respect to leadership, one that I have yet to discover within the literature is about leaders doing what they do most, dealing with the unexpected.

DEALING WITH THE UNEXPECTED

If one considers the notion of leadership as path making it is inevitable that one will encounter the unexpected, probably more frequently than when undertaking management or administrative roles. In my experience when one encounters the unexpected it is not *what* one does that matters but *how*. In each situation a multiplicity of options exists, each having a variety of repercussions, which ultimately impact on people. The effective leader works with staff to consider the implications of these impacts and agree decisions. The less effective leader makes decisions and informs staff of the impact. The findings from a study on clinical leadership suggested that this is how effective leaders were differentiated from the not so effective (Cook 2000).

Leadership and management

Covey (1989) refers to an emotional bank account to which it is very difficult to make deposits (leaders have to work hard to gain the respect of followers) but very easy to make withdrawals (leaders can lose that respect very quickly).

By motivation and inspiration, effective leaders can 'pull' staff along with them rather than 'pushing' from behind, which may be the inclination, especially when under pressure. This approach, along with genuine acknowledgement and recognition of the needs of staff, can increase performance significantly, and thus lead to improvement in patient/client care.

It is this leadership activity, rather than further, continuous organisational restructuring that is likely to have real impact on service delivery.

Having identified key aspects of administration, management and leadership it is apparent that a major aspect of all three areas is dealing and interacting with people. In the context of this chapter this means dealing with people in three main dimensions:

- people that one reports to, one's supervisor or line manager
- people that one supervises or provides line management to
- people that one works with, peers and colleagues.

Using the three terms 'mentorship', 'preceptorship' and 'clinical supervision' it is possible to align each of these terms to different aspects of the role:

- people that one reports to, one's supervisor or line manager – mentorship
- people that one supervises or provides line management to – preceptorship
- people that one works with, peers and colleagues – clinical supervision.

THE IMPORTANCE OF MENTORSHIP, PRECEPTORSHIP AND CLINICAL SUPERVISION AS A MANAGEMENT TOOL TO SUPPORT STAFF

Each of the three terms reflects aspects of a person's role within the workplace. This requires a brief understanding of role theory and Biddle (1979, p. 58) provides a succinct definition of role: '... those behaviours characteristic of one or more persons in context'. Biddle states that the definition encompasses four broad terms:

- behaviour
- person
- context
- characteristicness.

This suggests that we are in a dynamic state in relation to the roles that we undertake. The way that we adopt these roles depends upon our personality and the situations in which we find ourselves. It is important to understand that with such broad definitions there is no one right way of performing these roles; what is perhaps more important is to understand the broad principles and to adopt these principles as required of the context. This is not to suggest that acting out these roles is simple. Indeed, the three areas of mentorship, preceptorship and clinical supervision have the potential for complex and demanding situations. This is referred to as role conflict and can be seen in two main ways.

1. the definition of the role is ambiguous and expectations are not clear
2. conflict between the perceptions of the role and those demanded by the cultural context.

It is therefore important to know the expectations required of the role and the cultural environment in which one is undertaking the role. This has to be coupled with an understanding of the differences between these roles.

Mentoring

Mentoring has been in existence for many years, and stems from the world of politics and business (see Chapter Six). A mentor was generally linked to fostering and shaping successors within organisations. Mentors were seen to be critical for promotion by providing opportunities and information. This type of mentorship still survives and many readers will be able to think of one person that has been influential in their own career development. Collins (1983) identifies five criteria that should be satisfied to be considered a mentor and also identifies what a mentor is not (Box 5.1).

The literature abounds with the benefits of mentorship. These include sharing of ideas, increased satisfaction and productivity and the development of leadership, decision making and administrative skills (Beyer & Marshall 1981, Hamilton 1981, Chamings & Brown 1984).

Leadership and management

135

Box 5.1 Description of a mentor (after Collins 1983)

A mentor is:
- higher up the organisational ladder than the mentee
- an authority in their field
- influential
- interested in the growth and developments of the mentee
- willing to commit time and emotion to the relationship

A mentor is not:
- a pal
- on call for grievances and frustrations
- the exclusive mentor of the mentee
- someone who can be gracefully dismissed when no longer useful
- one's boss

It is also important to identify that there are drawbacks to mentorship. One such possibility is that the growth and development of the mentee is not fostered and a subservient role is encouraged and perpetuated by the mentor, which may result in exploitation. It is therefore important that both mentor and mentee review the relationship at periodic intervals to determine the suitability of continuation.

Based on research undertaken in nurse education (Cook 1998) the following points were deemed to be important by students of nursing and their ward supervisors for effective mentorship:

- The mentor knows the clinical area of the mentee. This does not have to be intimate knowledge of the actual clinical area, but an awareness of the broad circumstances is deemed to be important
- The mentor should themselves be respected within the care area and provide an effective environment in which others can care
- The mentor must be up to date, specifically so in respect to the changing policy context
- The mentor should be supportive without being directive; they should have an understanding of their own role and the expectations of the mentee
- The mentor should be willing to provide learning opportunities for the mentee and encourage the mentee to seek their own new learning opportunities.

Preceptorship

Preceptorship is variously defined, drawing on the work of the UKCC (1990). The aim of the role is to help newly qualifying nurses be supported to ease transition into professional practice from their student role into their qualified nurse's role. There seems to be a lack of rigorous evaluation of the process and outcomes in action, but anecdotal evidence suggests that when undertaken with serious commitment preceptorship has a positive outcome for both the new employee and the organisation.

The approach to preceptorship differs from organisation to organisation. As with mentorship a vital starting point is to understand the needs of the newly qualifying nurse, within the care context. A further important aspect of preceptorship is the selection of suitable staff to offer preceptorship. The UKCC (1993) recognised that preceptors require specific preparation for their role.

A debate that requires further attention is an allocation of time to undertake the preceptorship role within the normal working day. From personal experience many staff provide excellent preceptorship and this is often undertaken in their own time. Whilst this commitment to the nursing profession is to be applauded, it is important that leaders and managers convince resource allocators that investment in additional staffing hours to support such initiatives would improve both nursing care outcomes and help to recruit and retain valuable staff. Work being undertaken in the USA supports the view that investment in staff results in improved patient care and higher staff satisfaction (Aiken et al 2000).

In Australia preceptorship is being taken seriously with many nursing care providers offering extensive programmes to newly qualifying nurses, often linked to an academic award and involving rotation through various nursing specialty areas. Such programmes are also being offered throughout the UK as NHS trusts work hard to attract nurses to vacant posts.

Clinical supervision

The UKCC stated in its position paper on clinical supervision that:

> Clinical supervision brings practitioners and skilled supervisors together to reflect on practice. Supervision aims to identify solutions to problems, improve and increase understanding of professional issues. (UKCC 1996, p. 2)

Leadership and management

It is further stated that clinical supervision:

- is not a managerial control system
- is not the exercise of overt managerial responsibility or managerial supervision
- is not a system of formal individual performance review
- is not hierarchical in nature.

Clinical supervision is an important mechanism to 'help nurses function against a backdrop of constant change within health care' (Marrow et al 1998, p. 8). Research and empirical work into clinical supervision has been increasing, with much of the literature supporting its use. Various models exist and it is important to select an approach that suits individual circumstances. Marrow et al (1998) identify that to be successful clinical supervision requires six main elements to be addressed, as follows:

- *Commitment* – supervisors need to be committed to the concept of clinical supervision as it requires time and energy.
- *Training and development* – these are required for both parties; particularly important to attain is the skill of reflection.
- *Time* – as with mentorship, preceptorship clinical supervision requires allocated time to undertaken the role purposefully.
- *Ground rules* – these need to be clearly agreed and adherence checked at periodic intervals.
- *Reflection* – as mentioned earlier, reflection is an essential skill and should be used to promote problem solving. The potential for personal feelings to surface in a clinical supervision relationship should not be underestimated and both parties need to be aware of this and have access to a professional counselling service should this be required.
- *Support* – support is essential through any change process and it is inevitable that more support will be required at the early stages of the relationship.

The most important feature of clinical supervision is that it should enhance nursing care. It is therefore important at the outset to agree specific areas of attention and to agree mechanisms for monitoring these outcomes. In this way the benefit of investing in clinical supervision can be tied directly to improvement in care. This is not to negate the probable benefits in satisfaction on the part of nurses involved in clinical supervision, but a major reason for this investment is improved nursing care.

STRESS AS AN IMPORTANT POSITIVE INSTRUMENT TO ACHIEVE CHANGE

As identified earlier, the world of nursing and health care is a demanding and stressful environment. Earlier sections identified the importance of balancing the three aspects of administration, management and leadership. It was also identified that by working within a supportive environment through mentorship, preceptorship and clinical supervision, the negative impacts of this pressured environment can be dealt with in a positive way. This is explored further in Chapter Eight.

CONCLUSION

This chapter has identified that for health care provision to improve effective leaders and managers must ensure that support mechanisms are put in place for staff. Three such mechanisms have been described: preceptorship, mentorship and clinical supervision. This coupled with a review of the environmental factors in which care is provided should help promote an environment where care can be delivered to a high standard.

Practice checklist and discussion questions

Whilst undertaking the following exercises try not to feel guilty about where you could improve; instead note these points and celebrate the areas where you do well.

> ### Practice checklist
>
> - Do you know how the staff feel about the level of support they receive to their job? Try leading and managing by walking about. Take the time to ask staff, find out what three things you could do to help support them in their daily work. Take some time to collate the various responses and prioritise two actions over a month. How did staff react?
> - How much time do you seriously spend in focusing on patient care? Try to keep a diary just for a week; note how often you are really involved in decisions that impact on patient care. If this is less than you thought, what could you do differently?

Leadership and management

Discussion questions

- What work do you do in terms of administration, management and leadership, what could you do better or delegate?
- What support mechanisms do you employ or encourage for yourself or staff? Could these be improved?
- How do you deal with the unexpected? Could you deal with circumstances differently? What support and help could you offer others or need yourself?

References

Aiken L, Havens D S, Sloane D M 2000 Magnet nursing services recognition programme. Nursing Standard 14(25): 41–47

Allen D 2000 The NHS is in need of strong leadership. Nursing Standard 14(25): 25

Baggott R 1998 Health and health care in Britain, 2nd edn. Macmillan, London

Benton D 1997 Leading from the front: nursing leadership. Nursing Standard 11(37): 22–23

Beyer J E, Marshall J 1981 The interpersonal dimension of collegiality. Nursing Outlook 29: 662–665

Biddle B J 1979 Role theory expectations, identities and behaviours. Academic Press, London

Bolman L G, Deal T E 1991 Reframing organisations; artistry choice and leadership. Josey-Bass, San Francisco

Booth B 1995 Leading frights ... effective leaders. Nursing Times 91(23): 58

Burkitt I, Husband C, Mackenzie J et al 2000 Evaluating cognitive and affective processes in educational preparation for individualised care in pre and post registration education and practice. Final report to the ENB, Ethnicity and Social Policy Research Unit, University of Bradford

Capra F 1997 The web of life. Flamingo, London

Chamings P A, Brown B J 1984 The dean as mentor. Nursing and Health Care 5: 88–91

Collins N W 1983 Professional women and mentors. Prentice Hall, Englewood Cliffs, NJ

Cook M J 1998 Quality improvement through organisational improvement. Total Quality Management Special Issue, Proceedings of the 3rd World Congress for Total Quality Management. Business Excellence through Quality Culture 9: S35–37

Cook M J 1999 Improving care requires leadership in nursing. Nurse Education Today 19(4): 306–312

Cook M J 2000 Uncovering the attributes of effective clinical nurse leaders: a grounded theory approach. EdD thesis (unpublished), University of Lincolnshire and Humberside, Lincoln

Managing and supporting people

Connolly M 1997 The naked truth ... nursing leadership. Nursing Times 93(12): 27

Covey S 1989 The seven habits of highly effective people. Simon and Schuster, London

Cunningham G, Whitby E 1997 Power redistribution. Health Management September: 14–15

Dahlgaard J J, Larsen H Z, Norgaard A 1997 Leadership profiles in quality management. Total Quality Management 8(2&3): 516–530

Deming W E 1986 Out of the crisis. MIT Center for Advanced Engineering Study, Cambridge, MA

Department of Health 1997 The new NHS: modern, dependable. Department of Health, London

Department of Health 1998 A first class service: quality in the new NHS. Department of Health, London

Department of Health 1999 Making a difference: strengthening the nursing, midwifery and health visiting contribution to health and health care. Department of Health, London

Department of Health and Social Security 1983 National Health Service management enquiry (Griffiths Report). HMSO, London

Hamilton M W 1981 Mentorhood: a key to nursing leadership. Nursing Leadership 4: 4–13

Hulatt I 1995 A sad reflection. Nursing Standard 9(20): 22–23

Jarrold K 1998 A view from here: "servants and leaders". In: Martin S (ed.) The York Symposium on Health. 30th July, Department of Health Studies, University of York

Joiner B L 1994 Fourth generation management: the new business consciousness. McGraw Hill, New York

Maggs C 1996 Professors of nursing as clinicians and academics: is this the way forward? Nursing Times Research 1(2): 157–158

Marrow C E, Yaseen T, Cook M 1998 Caring together: clinical supervision. Royal College of Nursing (RCN) Update. Learning Unit 77. Nursing Standard 12(22)

Norman A 1995 Professional leadership in community nursing services. Health Visitor 8(1): 21–23

Porter-O'Grady T 1994 Whole systems shared governance: creating the seamless organisation. Nursing Economics. 12(4): 187–195

Rowden R 1995 Crisis? What crisis? Nursing Times 91(37): 50

Salvage J 1999 Speaking out ... supersisters ... clinical leadership. Nursing Times 95(21): 22

Sams D 1996 The development of leadership skills in clinical practice. Nursing Times 92(28): 37–39

Smith S 1997 The loneliness of a long-term leader. 12th National Ward Leaders' Conference, London, May 7–8. Nursing Times 93(12): 30–31

United Kingdom Central Council 1990 The report of the post registration education and practice project. UKCC, London

United Kingdom Central Council 1993 Registrar's Letter 1/1993. UKCC, London

United Kingdom Central Council 1996 Position statement on clinical supervision for nursing and health visiting. UKCC, London

Warner M, Langley M, Gould E, Picek A 1998 Healthcare futures 2010. Welsh Institute for Health and Social Care, Glamorgan

West-Burnham J 1998 The contribution of higher education to the development of educational leadership. Inaugural professorial lecture, University of Hull (unpublished)

Wheatley M 1994 Leadership and the new science: learning about organisations from an orderly universe. Berrett-Koehler, San Francisco

Williams S, Michie S, Pattani S 1998 Improving the health of the workforce – report on the partnership on the health of the NHS workforce. Nuffield Trust, London

Managing and supporting people

Leadership and quality:

partners in developing the service and staff

In this application Mullen provides an example of a quality framework to support the development of leadership and quality at every level in an organisation. The 'Baldrige' (NIST 2001) model describes several criteria that any organisation can use to improve overall performance, namely leadership, strategic planning, customer and market focus, information and analysis, human resources, process management and business results. The framework enabled professional cultural barriers to be overcome. It demonstrates again that the implementation of a systematic framework can provide a vehicle for change, at the same time allowing for individual approaches to implementation in teams. Equally important is the recognition of the education and training issues that can emerge and need to be addressed organisationally.

INTRODUCTION

The National Health Service (NHS) has always been committed to providing a professional service. However, a professional service does not always translate into a customer service. In the past few years there has been a recognition that these two approaches, whilst not mutually exclusive, can lead to different experiences for patients. Those in the NHS know that they need to focus more on the patient and to do this we need to change from a professionally orientated service to a more customer orientated service. In the process of doing this one organisation I worked in started to consider a total quality management model called 'Baldrige' which at that time was relatively unknown. The 'interest' was started at the top, by the chief executive, which was vital if this approach was to have any chance of succeeding. Why? The chief executive, like a ward sister/charge nurse,

143

'sets the culture' of an organisation through their leadership and beliefs about 'how' things are done.

WHAT IS BALDRIGE?

The Baldrige framework was formally established in the USA in 1987 and originated out of the need to raise the importance of quality for achieving better business results. Malcolm Baldrige was Secretary of Commerce from 1981 and championed the initiative until he died in a road accident in 1987. In recognition of his commitment they decided to name the award in his honour. The Malcolm Baldrige National Quality Award was established to alert senior managers to the need for putting quality as the key driver and to reward those organisations that excelled in having successful quality systems in place.

The Baldrige system and criteria

The Baldrige framework has seven key criteria with four key elements:

1. *Driver* – senior executive leadership is a central role
2. *System* – a whole systems thinking to the organisation's processes that is documented and well managed
3. *Measures of progress* – established performance measures that inform and activate the continuous improvement process
4. *Goals* – results, both non-financial and financial.

The 'Baldrige' experience

So how did we do it? We took our time! Everyone knows how busy staff are in the NHS, running about 'doing their best under difficult circumstances'. The last thing that staff wanted to hear was about another 'quality project' that would be the 'in thing' for about 4 months, which would then disappear into the abyss of history as yet another 'one-off, flavour of the month'! The nursing director often has the lead for quality and therefore as the director of nursing and quality I had the responsibility of developing a quality strategy for the trust. The problem is that quality was viewed as another 'add on' thing to do and was not thought of as central to the job in hand. This is where the story begins.

The journey

The Baldrige framework provided the opportunity to redraw the picture about how a quality model can be used in everyday practice rather than as a 'one-off, quick fix'. Initially we undertook several training sessions for directorates and staff at all levels to help staff understand how the approach can help them, their staff and their service on a daily basis. The Baldrige framework is a whole systems approach based on the principles of total quality management. The framework provides you with a toolkit for putting the principles into action. This is usually what NHS staff like – action! Another key attraction to the model is that it can be as simple or as complicated as you like. Therefore all levels and abilities of staff can 'have a go'. It is based on common sense, it gives staff ownership of the process and is developmental along the way.

During the implementation of Baldrige, we soon learnt that, because the model originated in America, some of the 'language' was difficult to translate into 'English'. As a consequence, after 12 months we transferred over to the European version (the European Organisational Excellence Model) which has the same approach and principles but is written in 'English'. The important thing was to get staff involved across all disciplines and across all services.

One of the main criteria of the framework is leadership, without which the system will fail. The sisters/charge nurses on wards/departments are key 'leaders' in the NHS and are central to creating the culture at ward/departmental level. We therefore encouraged the sisters/charge nurses to be involved in using the framework as a way of working. It is also important to get the support of the line managers, as they need to facilitate staff in taking actions as a consequence of using the framework. Once the staff had bought the ticket the rest was about support and facilitation.

The Baldrige framework in action

In all organisations 're-engineering' – often a fancy word for restructuring – is a common feature. One of the departments that had re-engineered involved a large group of professionals from different backgrounds who had come together in one management unit. This involved physiotherapists, chiropodists, occupational therapists, dietitians and speech therapists. This was not an easy quest as they were all fiercely independent and did not particularly see the benefit of being managed together within one unit. The manager had attended several sessions on the Baldrige/European framework and decided to try to use the framework as a process for change management. This was a brave step but after 18 months the department had reorganised itself and had developed systems for working together as one unit, much to the staff's surprise. The model helped them to develop and streamline their systems for recruiting staff, measuring staff satisfaction, measuring patient satisfaction and for developing their own staff appraisal system. This was quite amazing as every group had previously had different ways of doing

145

all these things. The outcome of this success was that they developed a term for solving problems within their own unit: 'If something needs fixing, let's Baldrige it'. A few months later this unit started to write all their business plans using the model. They also developed a framework for undertaking a self-assessment of their service every year using the model as their measure of continuous improvement. This is leadership in action as all staff are involved and the manager even took the risk of asking the staff to evaluate her performance!

Another example is amongst ward sisters/charge nurses, from different areas, who had a mutual problem about record keeping. The sisters got together from A&E, mental health and one of the medical wards and, using the framework, they assessed the problem and prioritised the actions for improving this important area. An audit tool was developed and formed part of an annual cycle of evaluation and self-assessment. A spin-off from this was that the group became very good friends, despite being from very different services. They now have regular social evenings, which proves that learning together can be fun as well as hard work!

USING QUALITY AS A MODEL FOR DEVELOPMENTAL LEARNING

In the process of using the framework it became clear that once staff began using the model it highlighted that ward staff in particular needed some development and support. These included such things as writing a business plan, writing a project plan, problem solving, motivating staff and implementing change. These issues were fed into the training and development programme within the trust and began to form part of an individual's personal development plan. The process also enabled sisters/charge nurses to use a whole systems approach to their service and provided them with a framework for measuring their performance. This also provided the staff with a measurement tool to assess their service for continuous improvement performance on an annual basis. It is not an easy option but in the long run it is proactive, applicable anywhere, measurable and interactive.

What the staff said

The staff involved in the process said many things, not all of which I can capture in this small section but below are some of the feelings and benefits that staff had about using the model:

- 'At first I wasn't sure I would understand it but when the penny dropped I thought it was great.'
- 'It helped me see the whole thing, not just my bit.'

- 'It was hard work but I think in the end it is worth it as I understand my role better.'
- 'It gave me a way of finding out what the real cause of the problem was.'
- 'It helped me prioritise as there is always too much to do and I never could decide which to do first so I usually ended up trying to do it all and never finished anything. This way I knew which was the most important and did that first without worrying about the others.'
- 'My boss tried to be the leader in the project but was not very good at it because she did not know the service as well as I do so in the end she handed over the project lead to me. It gave me a feeling of value and the boss really appreciates what we do now.'
- 'Quality isn't easy but it is worth it in the end.'
- 'I learnt such a lot about my staff and myself. It was really good as well as hard work.'

Why should you use it?

We have now a White Paper *A First Class Service* (DoH 1998) that is committed to the quality of service and clinical care that we provide to our patients. The NHS is a busy environment and we do not have time to treat quality as 'an added extra'. The only way that we can successfully improve our service and quality is to integrate quality into everything we do. This is one model for doing that. The model has been used successfully in industry, schools and the police service both in the UK and in Europe. The challenge to all professionals is to recognise the changing expectations and knowledge base of our patients, families and friends. Nursing is a main player in the delivery of care. Nurses can and should be the ones leading the way on quality of patient care. This model will provide a way for leaders in care to assess their service and measure their journey towards excellence. If your trust has a total quality management philosophy then you are half-way there. All it would take for the next step is for you to buy the ticket and take the journey. The words are easy – it is the action that makes it real.

References

Department of Health 1998 A first class service: quality in the new NHS. Department of Health, London

NIST 2001 Frequently asked questions and answers about the Malcolm Baldrige National Quality Award. Fact sheet from the National Institute of Standards and Technology: http://www.quality.nist.gov/

Leadership and quality: partners in developing the service and staff

Application 5:2

Tracy Packer

Developing new roles:

learning from a nurse consultant

Using her experience in her role as a nurse consultant, Packer discusses key learning points to share with those who are in the role currently, or who may aspire to achieving such a role in the future.

INTRODUCTION

The Nurse Consultant in Dementia Care post came into being at North Bristol NHS Trust in April 2000, one of the first in the country to take up the new nurse consultant role as a key part of the government's modernisation programme. This unique role remains grounded within the service provided by those working on the acute wards of the Medical Directorate of a large general teaching hospital. The postholder has responsibility for the strategic development of care to people with dementia on 27 units across three hospital sites, and must do this in conjunction with an unusual but well-established and skilled team of an 18-bed acute unit for people with dementia also provided within the auspices of the Medical Directorate.

In order to achieve this the nurse consultant must collaborate with medical staff, allied health professionals and other specialist teams across the Trust, particularly from within the neurology, orthopaedic and palliative care units, along with medical and nursing staff and other professionals from within the psychiatry of old age service provided by a neighbouring Mental Healthcare Trust. Communication and collaboration with independent, voluntary and social service organisations within the Trust region and beyond is also considered an essential part of the role. The postholder is professionally accountable to the Director of Nursing, and clinically accountable to the Medical Directorate Head of Nursing and the Clinical Director who is a consultant physician.

AN OVERVIEW OF THE JOB DESCRIPTION

The guidelines for the creation of nurse consultant posts (DoH 1999) state clearly that they must contain four key elements. These were strictly adhered to when drawing up the job description for the North Bristol NHS Trust proposal. These key elements were:

- Expert practice
- Professional leadership and consultancy
- Education, training and development
- Practice and service development.

The day-to-day running of the role does not of course divide neatly into each of these four elements, although attempting this in order to justify one's activity could be an easy trap to fall into. It has been more helpful to take a flexible position whereby all of the necessary elements could potentially be contained in each of the tasks that are undertaken. A particular element may naturally dominate at different times, depending on the emphasis and progress of an initiative. However, in ideal circumstances the postholder will be considering each element and its potential place in every development with which they become involved.

DEFINING 'CLINICAL PRACTICE'

Keeping 'experienced nurses by the bedside' for at least 50% of their time has been a key soundbite in the government media campaign to promote the nurse consultant initiative. Indeed, the maintenance of clinical contact is a core concept and many members of the public have been able to identify with this ideal. In practice, however, this is not as straightforward as it first sounds.

The North Bristol post has stipulated that the ratio of clinical to non-clinical time in post should be approximately 60:40, which (on paper), is more optimistic than the government's predictions of 50:50. However, how can clinical practice be defined for this purpose? Spending several hours on a unit, trying to piece together the intricacies of the actions of a person with dementia who is challenging the team, must include in-depth conversations with the nurses, the medical staff and other members of the multidisciplinary team along with a review of all the case notes. It often includes meeting the relatives and more importantly, always involves spending time with the person concerned. Whilst up to 25% of this time may involve direct patient contact, the other 75% of this input provides the opportunity for a comprehensive review and assessment of what is or isn't happening. The nurse consultant may well be applying their expertise in the dementia field and their privileged 'helicopter view' of the situation in order to suggest a way forward, but this remaining

Developing new roles: learning from a nurse consultant

time cannot strictly be described as 'direct nursing care'. However, it is (I would argue) relevant clinical practice, the effect of which may make a lasting impact upon the experience of care by the person with dementia, and contribute to the understanding of needs required by the ward team and/or family carers.

If there is little doubt that interventions such as those described above should be classed as clinical practice, what about the use of dementia care mapping (DCM)? DCM is an observational tool that is used to try to establish the level of wellbeing a person with dementia is experiencing in a given care environment (Kitwood & Bredin 1992, Brooker 1995). Although it was not originally conceived for use on acute admissions units (it has been an effective tool on assessment and continuing care units; Brooker & Payne 1995, Wilkinson 1995, Williams & Rees 1995), the observational process and particular aspects of the methodology provide an opportunity to see the environment and the person with dementia in it, from a completely different perspective of that of the care staff. For this reason it is ideal to use as a staff development and learning tool even within the acute sector. The observers, throughout the many hours of the process, generally have no direct patient contact, but the changes that are often made to care plans as a result of DCM can have tremendous clinical benefit. This is a tool that:

- needs a skilled facilitator
- takes place in the direct care environment with all the ensuing
· ethical considerations, alongside direct care staff
- can make an important contribution to individual care planning.

Can this be described as clinical practice or not?

I have argued, of course, that it is. However, I have increasingly become aware that this is a role-specific query that can be difficult to explain to those from outside the field, particularly because working at the interface of people who have dementia and the professionals who care for them, depends upon complex communication skills and increased awareness of more nebulous concepts such as co-dependency, rather than more visible levels of technical expertise or the ability to carry out a complex medical task. (Although these too have their place, and should not be too easily dismissed.) For every area of care in which nurse consultants are based, there will undoubtedly be similar examples of difficulty in justifying specific interventions because it is not possible to categorise them neatly within the 'clinical practice' box. The irony, I have come to realise, is that everything I do ultimately aims to influence and improve clinical practice, sometimes by my direct intervention in an immediate care process, but more often through working to improve the confidence and the competence of those around me. The realisation that I can't do everything myself just because I know how it is done has, at times, been a difficult and (on occasion) painful lesson to learn. When I am asked about the ratio of time spent in 'clinical practice' I have, 3 years on, become confident in the knowledge that indeed 60% of my time is spent in this way. I can justify my definition of 'clinical practice' because I have the confidence and understanding of the complexity of the role to do so. In truth, if the definition as understood by most people (and probably most politicians) were applied – i.e. 'direct care delivery to a patient in a clinical setting' – I would have to say it is currently about 30% which is, I would argue, entirely appropriate.

Not unreasonably, many people are concerned that in time, the pressure on nurse consultants to take part in external consultancy, writing for publication, facilitating training programmes and delivering conference presentations will soon 'swallow up' the time available for direct care. These are valid concerns, but it is important not to overlook the vital part these aspects of the role have to play in disseminating good practice, exposing services to new ways of thinking and providing staff with a broader range of perspectives and expectations with which to tackle complex needs. These too provide a perhaps unforeseen benefit associated with being a positive role model. As my own role has evolved with many such opportunities being made available to me, staff in North Bristol NHS Trust have remained very positive and keen to collaborate in experiences that also give them the opportunity to share their good practice with others outside the service, speak at conferences, become involved in a range of teaching opportunities and write up their own work for publication. These are opportunities not previously sourced so readily within the clinical areas, providing mentorship for an additional raft of personal development opportunities for nurses and their colleagues in other professions who will lead and develop the services of the future. The value of this input cannot be understated.

For those considering taking on a similar role, or who are thinking of including a nurse consultant in their team, the following advice may be helpful.

HAVE A VISION, AND HOLD ON TO IT

Three years after the introduction of nurse consultant roles, I can still safely say that many people (including nurses) still do not know quite what to expect from them. Many nurses, along with other professional colleagues, still have not come into contact with a nurse consultant in their everyday clinical work, nor have many members of the public been able to make sense of 'where in the NHS hierarchy' nurse consultants fit. This is the everyday reality of the nurse consultant role, primarily because most nurses and other health and social care professions have not been exposed to colleagues who have worked at this level whilst also maintaining a strong clinical link. This could be perceived as a major advantage because, even now, nobody has any fixed notion about what nurse consultants should or should not be doing, as long as it can be defined against the original Department of Health guidelines. This continues to provide a tremendous opportunity for imaginative and unique role development across specialty and organisational boundaries.

Care should always be taken in the early stages of the development of a new nurse consultant post, and should continue long after the post has been recruited into. It is becoming increasingly clear that the absence of a nursing vision regarding these posts can translate into nurse consultants becoming no more than glorified clinical specialists, trying to meet the agenda of every clinician and manager in their service. Whilst expertise and clinical credibility within a defined specialist area may very much be a part of what makes a good nurse consultant, those appointed in these early years have a very real responsibility to ensure that these roles contribute directly to the dynamic evolution of the nursing profession as a whole. They have been, and should continue to be, an important part of a bigger template that should enable the profession to expand far beyond the limitations previously experienced, seizing this opportunity to actively define that which follows.

DON'T DENY THE POLITICS

North Bristol NHS Trust was already looking at developing a senior nursing role of this nature before the nurse consultant role was outlined by the Department of Health. In our case, politicisation was just the leverage we required for making the case for creating such a role and generating the funding to support it. Equally, the Royal College of Nursing and the Nursing and Midwifery Council (previously the UKCC) had been developing frameworks for 'expert' leadership roles within nursing for some years prior to their announcement, and there must have been some delight at those early proclamations. Whilst it would be foolish to try to erase the current political agenda from any discussions about the role of the nurse consultant, only time will tell whether or not the current government modernisation programme (of which the development of such roles has played a crucial part) has indeed been a valid intervention. In the meantime, many health and social care professionals have viewed politicisation of nurse consultant posts with a great deal of scepticism. By acknowledging the context and influence of the political agenda in the short term, nurse leaders and managers will put themselves in a better position to expand on the longer term development possibilities for the nursing profession.

For me, this approach has proven to be very fruitful. Recognising the initial political resonance in a team discussion of the nurse consultant role, and validating the feelings that inevitably transpire, has actually 'freed up' those concerned for enthusiastic discussion and debate about what can be gained by having such a role in place. This has, in turn, unlocked real opportunities for innovative, multidisciplinary working. Once a nurse consultant can establish professional credibility, early cynicism about politicisation soon passes.

BEWARE OF CAST-OFF ROLES

Think carefully before *automatically* taking on quasi-medical roles, or any other roles already in existence that have apparent kudos attributed to them. There is a danger that this could happen in the early months of a nurse consultant appointment, particularly in an environment where very few people are certain about how the role will 'shape up' in the long term. Whilst some quasi-medical tasks certainly could have a place within a nurse consultant role, it is important that these do not supersede the development and evaluation of important but undervalued nursing interventions. It is also important to be wary of roles that other professionals would rather relinquish in order to concentrate on their other work. Such opportunities may indeed provide genuine scope for a truly innovative service development, but it is important to review the possibilities in the light of the overall aims and objectives of the nurse consultant role. It is also important to avoid becoming 'pigeon-holed'.

There is no doubt that trying to develop these new posts beyond the sometimes limited expectations of others may at times make life uncomfortable for the postholder. It is important to realise that others often define nurse consultants in relationship to what they themselves feel they gain out of their working relationship with you. This can lead to many different and sometimes unrealistic expectations, no genuine understanding of what you really do, and a failure to recognise that you cannot not be 'all things to all people'. It is tempting to try to keep 'all of the people happy all of the time', but this flies in the face of good leadership and can cause a high level of fragmentation in your working life. If there is to be real progress in developing nursing as a profession, it is essential that these new roles really do rise above the mediocre.

PROGRESSING THE NURSE CONSULTANT ROLE – KEY LEARNING POINTS

Nurse consultants should:

● Take the importance of being a positive role model very seriously, not only for other nurses, but also as a representative to other disciplines of all that nurses can aspire to be. This matters as much when dealing with differences of opinion as when engaged in expert practice.

- Remember that this role is much more than the sum of a clinical caseload. Nurse consultants need to develop *people* if they are to successfully develop *services,* thus emphasising the need to empower those around them. The 'supernurse' analogy much loved by the media is all very well, but saving the day is only good for the ego of the person doing the saving and gives everyone else a message that they are somehow incapable of making a difference. This can never be a recipe for a positive learning environment, nor for creative service development.

- Devise extensive networks at all levels *within* the employing organisation. External networking is valid in its own right, but even the most impressive external network will not always be able to help in the day-to-day practical and clinical dilemmas that may arise in the workplace. The value of good relationships with administrative, portering, catering and reception staff amongst others should never be taken for granted.

- Take a course in media and presentation skills. The local interest in nurse consultants alone can generate numerous photo opportunities, newspaper and radio interviews and television coverage, but even without this it can contribute to a more confident delivery during conference presentations and other public speaking events. Preparation of this kind may also become useful at a later date when a nurse-led development requires (as well as generates) a little media coverage to help it along!

- Identify a national network of professional peers working in a similar field who could become a safe source of support and topical information exchange; always be proactive in staying in touch with them. (These individuals should come from a variety of professional backgrounds to maximise your exposure to different perspectives in your particular field of interest.)

- Get an external mentor. This person does not necessarily have to be another nurse, but they must be able to challenge the postholder and help them to recognise their weaknesses as well as develop their strengths.

CONCLUSION

The nurse consultant role provides a significant opportunity to promote key elements of expert nursing skills, at a time when many nurses are finding it difficult to define just what these may be. Additionally, nurse consultants must play a significant part in the development of clinical nurses who are creative, reflective, articulate and willing to promote their work to anyone who will listen. There

Managing and supporting people

has never been a better time for the nursing profession to take an imaginative and active role in the development and validation of its own professional identity.

References

Brooker D 1995 Looking at them, looking at me: a review of observational studies into the quality of institutional care for elderly people with dementia. Journal of Mental Health 4: 145–156

Brooker D, Payne M 1995 Auditing outcomes of care in in-patient and day patient settings using dementia care mapping. Can it be done? PSIGE Newsletter 51: 18–22

Department of Health 1999 Nurse consultant posts. Health Service Circular. Department of Health, London

Kitwood T, Bredin K 1992 A new approach to the evaluation of dementia care. Journal of Advances in Health and Nursing Care 1(5): 41–60

Wilkinson A M 1995 Dementia care mapping: a pilot study of its implementation in a psychogeriatric service. International Journal of Geriatric Psychiatry 8: 1027–1029

Williams J, Rees J 1995 The use of 'dementia care mapping' as a method of evaluating care received by patients with dementia: an initiative to improve quality of life. Journal of Advanced Nursing 25: 316–323

Further reading

Manley K 1995 A conceptual framework for advanced practice: an action research project operationalizing an advanced practitioner/consultant nurse role. Journal of Clinical Nursing 6: 179–190

Manley K 2000 Organisational culture and consultant nurse outcomes: Part 1, organisational culture. Nursing Standard 14: 36

Manley K 2000 Organisational culture and consultant nurse outcomes: Part 2, nurse outcomes. Nursing Standard 14: 37

Manley K, Garbett R 2000 Paying Peter and Paul: reconciling concepts of expertise with competency for a clinical career structure. Journal of Clinical Nursing 9: 347–359

Packer T 2001 Acute Care Series Part 1: A nurse consultant in dementia care. Signpost 5(3): 19–22

Packer T 2001 Acute Care Series Part 2: Acute sector care for people with dementia: time to get our heads out of the sand. Signpost 5(4): 33–36

Developing new roles: learning from a nurse consultant

Section Three

MANAGING SELF – MAKING IT WORK FOR YOU

OVERVIEW

The first two sections of this book have concentrated on the global and organisational perspectives that must be addressed by managers and leaders when seeking to get the best out of people and thus strive towards high quality service provision.

Section Three addresses how you, as an individual, can ensure you have the skills and knowledge to make the system work for you as well as enabling you to work to your full capacity within the organisation. It stresses the responsibility to structure and manage the processes of self-development is your own, and whilst it may be helpful to seek out the views and support of others, finally the buck rests with you. You too have a responsibility to ensure your development complements the direction of the organisation, and also, in the case of clinical professionals, that you meet the requirements of your professional body.

Mentorship is a word that is used to describe many relationships, and often different professional groups use the term in different ways. This can be confusing so it is timely to comment here on how this section is interpreting the term. Mentorship in this context describes a relationship between two

157

OVERVIEW

people that is aimed at helping one or both of them to achieve personal growth and/or career development. Engaging in such a relationship enables individuals to test out ideas and think through options in a safe environment, some (virtual or actual) distance from the workplace.

Whilst personal and career development is not just about changing jobs, most of us will seek to do so at some stage in our professional life. There are ways that enable us to sell ourselves in a positive light, and therefore the important skills of curriculum vitae preparation and interview techniques are included here to help you achieve your objectives.

Having a balance in life is important too, and here you will find ideas to consider in helping you do just that, by offering suggestions to manage stressful situations effectively and constructively, and to help you maintain a healthy lifestyle.

Chapter **Six**

Mentoring in the workplace:

a process of growth and development

Julie Hyde

- The roots of mentorship
- Benefiting from mentorship
- Lifelong learning
- The mentorship relationship
- Characteristics of a mentor

- Responsibilities of the mentee
- Choosing a mentor
- Exploring the mentor/mentee relationship
- Focused mentoring

OVERVIEW

In this chapter Hyde outlines the history of the role of the mentor, and discusses some ways in which the role may be applied in the workplace. She points out that an effective mentoring process can be of value to the organisation as well as the individual as it is one way of developing staff, thus enabling them to make an organisational contribution. Each partner in the mentorship relationship has responsibilities, and these are outlined in the chapter. This is true also for other helping relationships, such as clinical supervision and clinical mentorship.

Six Steps to **Effective Management**

THE CONTRIBUTION OF MENTORING IN THE CONTEXT OF HEALTH CARE

Mentoring, as a description of a process, has long been part of the culture in the health care industry. The interpretation of the term 'mentor' has been one which has been open to debate. Within the health care sectors, and particularly within the nursing profession, originally the term 'mentor' was used to describe an individual who had responsibility for teaching, assessing and supporting a more junior member of staff (Conway 1998, Hyde 1988a, 1988b). This role was closely linked with the student status of the junior staff member and the requirement to achieve certain educational goals as part of the process of achieving a licence to practise.

There is nevertheless a core scheme of things – a kind of 'hierarchy of mentorship' – which serves here to demonstrate the breadth and depth of the potential of mentorship as a process. This is represented in Figure 6.1.

Over the past 15 years a plethora of terms and labels has emerged in health care speak in relation to supporting staff (both qualified and unqualified) in the clinical workplace. One which has gained ground, yet still seems to lack clarity, is *clinical supervision*. This process is widely used in the nursing profession, and often the terms 'clinical supervisor' and 'mentor' are used interchangeably. This results in confusion as mentorship is not unique

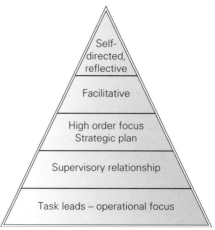

Figure 6.1 Hierarchy of mentorship support

Managing self – making it work for you

to health care. However, the skills inherent in both processes are similar and transferable, so how the process is *described* is less important, providing that clarity between those in the relationship exists.

It is useful to consider first a range of working definitions. This is not claimed to be the definitive of descriptors, but for clarity it is a helpful starting place.

Clinical supervision

Clinical supervision most usually describes a process of peer support whereby one health professional assists and supports another health professional (not necessarily of the same discipline) to reflect upon personal practice, either in general terms or in relation to a particular scenario. There is no intention within that relationship to work within a power or hierarchical framework, nor should the content of the discussions be used in a disciplinary way. It is not necessary that the clinical supervisor should work in the same organisation as the supervisee, but in practice this is often the case for pragmatic reasons. However, this proximity can have its problems as individuals may feel inhibited in their discussion, being aware that details of the context and the interpersonal relationships are well known to both parties and that hidden agendas may emerge.

Clinical mentorship

Clinical mentorship is a term used to describe the relationship between an expert practitioner within an area of practice and a person who is new to that area. Most often this is a relationship between a qualified professional and a 'student professional' and that relationship often embraces the tripartite role of teacher, assessor and critical friend. The term 'preceptorship' gained some popularity in the 1990s, and most often was used to describe the support a newly qualified health professional might receive in the first 6 months or so after first registration to facilitate the closure of the theory/practice gap. As the pressures on the service have increased steadily, the formalised preceptorship role has been marginalised and the processes of support adsorbed into the embrace of clinical supervision.

Mentoring in the workplace

161

THE ROOTS OF MENTORSHIP

As with many concepts of learning and personal growth, mentorship was first defined by the ancients Greeks via their mythology. The eponymous Mentor was friend of King Odysseus, who, prior to going away at war, asked Mentor to be support and companion to his son Telemachus. This role of wise counsellor has been a theme in many other places in literature and the Arts. Shakespeare used the relationship model (e.g. Bassanio and Antonio). More recently Star Wars films and the Harry Potter series have outlined the value of a young person seeking, or being given, wise counsel. The Prince of Wales has talked openly about the value of his friendship and mentorship relationship with Laurens Van Der Post.

The examples above describe relationships which are formalised and explicit in their nature. However, mentorship does not always have to be like that. Readers may be able immediately to think about an individual who, for them, has been an inspiration, a role model through a more informal relationship.

Gibb (2002, p. 271) suggests that there are three contexts to mentorship and from those he suggests that a number of themes emerge which impact on the individual's (i.e. mentee's) development (Box 6.1). All these themes have resonance in the context of health care today. A 'wise counsellor' may be able to play an active role in enabling an individual to 'achieve power' through either knowledge or introductions.

The master/apprentice relationship (sometimes described as 'sitting next to Nellie') was one that for many years served as a model for the training of nurses. As this is no longer applicable as nurses now are prepared within the higher education sector, the

Managing self – making it work for you

BOX 6.1 The three contexts of mentorship (adapted from Gibb 2002)

Context of mentorship	Emerging themes
Classical mythology	Role of 'wise counsel' Achievement of power
Craft guilds	Master/apprentice relationship and regulation of the crafts
Humanistic psychology	Transitions, helping processes, self-development in adults

role of the 'clinical mentor' has been outlined to support the students when they are working in the clinical areas.

The third context suggested by Gibb is focused on helping processes, with the individual taking responsibility for personal development, ideally with support, and this too is a model used in health care.

WHO BENEFITS FROM MENTORSHIP?

In this chapter, the term 'mentorship' will be defined in broader terms, to indicate and describe a process (whatever it might be called in different contexts) which supports and directs individuals, either singly or in groups, to develop their expertise and aspirations within any professional framework, and within a framework of lifelong learning. However, mentorship as a process should benefit not only the individual, but also the organisation in which the individual works; in addition, it should have a benefit for the mentor. In the context of this chapter, it is assumed that individuals are using the processes of mentorship to enhance their own professional development within their own career parameters. Indubitably the processes of mentorship can be used purely in personal self-development, perhaps after an illness or other traumatic life event, but the application of these processes is different, and is outside the remit of this chapter.

LIFELONG LEARNING

The concept of lifelong learning within the context of health care and in society in general is one which has reached significant prominence since the change of government in May 1997. This new administration has published a number of documents which embrace this concept. Pertinent to health care professionals are:

- the English White Paper *The New NHS: Modern, Dependable* (DoH 1997)
- the consultation document *A First Class Service: Quality in the New NHS* (DoH 1998a)
- the Health Service Circular *Working Together: Securing a Quality Workforce for the NHS* (DoH 1998b).

Building on these, *The NHS Plan: A Plan for Investment, A Plan for Reform* (DoH 2000) and *Shifting the Balance of Power in the NHS*

Mentoring in the workplace

(DoH 2001a) take forward the thrust that the wellbeing of the NHS and partner agencies depends on the currency and professionalism of the staff. Thus, within all these documents, there is an overt requirement for professionals to take a proactive approach to personal development and lifelong learning, as their own growth and development will contribute to the overall growth and development of the organisation, and thus to quality of service provision for its users. Lifelong learning can therefore be seen as a framework partnership between the individual and the workplace, and in this partnership the role of the mentor is an important one.

Government has on many occasions spoken out about its belief in the importance of effective leadership in achieving high quality health care for the public (see Ch. 5) and absent or ineffective leadership has been highlighted in some recent debates, for example *The Bristol Inquiry* (DoH 2001b). Leadership is open to all as it is not tied to a given role or position. To develop an individual's leadership skills and attributes, the role of a mentor has a great deal to offer.

LOOKING AHEAD

As an individual's career progresses, the focus on development needs becomes more specific. It becomes much less appropriate and/or usual for a need to be met by attending a formal course of education. More likely the need will be met by the individual reaching into past professional experience and transferring skills and experiences to the new world.

A number of writers asserts that mentorship is a particularly valuable and appropriate technique to apply in an environment of continuous change or instability (Hay 1995, Conway 1998, Clutterbuck & Megginson 1999, Whittaker & Cartwright 2000). This is particularly relevant in the NHS today, where, over the past 15 years, organisations, professions and individuals have witnessed enormous and far-reaching change, reputed to be the most significant at macro level since the instigation of the NHS in 1948.

The active process of mentorship can assist in the stabilisation of the organisation. At a micro level, change requires individuals to continually, and usually rapidly, adapt and practise in a number of circumstances and contexts, some of which may be new to them, new altogether (i.e. 'leading edge'), relatively permanent or highly transitory, and often not thought through at strategic level (i.e. 'knee-jerk' policy). Given the purpose and business of health care, to perform at less than optimum may have disastrous effects, and thus the stakes are high. In a context such as this, the role of a mentor is valuable. Unlike the requirements of the clinical supervision partnership, the mentor is an individual of significantly more experience than the mentee, and thus may be able to contribute both knowledge and a safe sounding board for reflection on any key decisions mentees may need to take.

This 'collective wisdom' suffered significant culling in the reforms of the internal market when the organisational cultures of competition and public sector health care were brought together. Fresh chief executives brought in their own executive boards and senior teams, and many of those who carried the organisations' history and memory left the service. Youth culture impacted on management styles, as fast track promotion took over from the culture of 'serving one's time for promotion'. With hindsight it can be reported that the fast turnover of chief executives, and inevitably some of their teams, resulted in decisions being made which had been tried (and not worked) before; in short there was a great deal of reinventing of wheels!

MENTORSHIP APPLIED

The mentorship relationship

In more recent years, the NHS has recognised the value of and the need to offer a formalised structure of mentorship to senior members of staff from both the clinical disciplines and those in management professions.

In the early 1990s the NHS Women's Unit was devised to help to balance out the number of men and women in top health care jobs, and this used the process of formalised mentorship. The King's Fund has a long history of providing development opportunities, and this scheme too recognises the contribution of the mentor.

Conway (1998, p. 93) describes a project in the (then) South West Thames Regional Health Authority which in 1991 introduced a mentoring scheme for G grade nurses (middle managers) within the region. The programme was designed to:

- be a positive and stimulating experience for all
- break down occupational barriers
- help each individual to grow both personally and professionally.

Mentoring in the workplace

This scheme recognised the power of the role model in the mentoring relationship. Clutterbuck & Megginson (1999) suggest that the role model component of mentoring is an important one. They suggest a 'model of mentoring role modelling' (p. 143) and this is described in Table 6.1.

Mentoring is an interactive, eclectic process. Both its power and effect are within the relationship between mentor and mentee. Some elements of the change management process are brought to

Table 6.1 A model of role modelling in mentoring relationships

Stage	Features	To move on
Acceptive awareness	Based on reputation, observation from a distance; recognizing role model as source of learning	Seeking out the mentor or being sought out
Admiration	Development of regard based on the role model's values, impact and (sometimes) interest in mentee	Dissatisfaction with aspects of oneself, which the mentor appears to have mastered
Adaptation	Conscious and unconscious process of change to adopt role model's behaviour, ways of thinking, values	Tune in to the mentor's behaviours, ideas, strategies, motives; commit to personal change
Advancement	Integrate mentor's mental models with one's own; practise new behaviour and observe results	Step back and look at the mentor more critically
Astute awareness	Mature evaluation of the role model – warts and all; reassert and also develop own values and mental models	Seek new sources of learning/role models; become more selective in distinguishing what to accept/reject

From Mentoring Executives and Directors by Clutterbuck & Megginson. Reprinted by permission of Elsevier Ltd the role of the mentor, as sometimes (though not always) the mentor may take the role of change agent, supporting the mentee through the processes (either chosen by or forced upon the mentee) of change. Chapter Three explores this more fully.

Mentoring is most usually delivered within a one-to-one relationship, but the basic principles of mentorship in any context or theme (see Box 6.1) can be applied in a multimentoring framework, often devised specifically to support and develop those undertaking a particular professional role. This fits within the framework of the mentoring model of *developmental alliance* described by Julie Hay (1995, p. 3). She defines a *developmental alliance* as:

> A relation between equals in which one or more of those involved is enabled to:
>
> ● Increase awareness
> ● Identify alternative and initiate action to
> ● Develop themselves.
>
> (Hay 1995, p. 3)

Hay's reference to 'equals' captures the fact that there may be several people within a mentoring relationship, and they are equal in value, even though their experiences may be different. It should be noted too that Hay's work was carried out in the USA where the idea of 'self-help groups' is more developed than it is in the UK. Interestingly, Hay's module of 'developmental alliance' is more like the model of clinical supervision used by some health professionals, using the collective knowledge to either solve a problem or move forward in practice.

This highlights the confusion that might arise as a result of differing terminology and semantics. In general, there seems to be a number of issues which characterise and affect the process and style of the mentoring relationship. These can be displayed simply within a continuum as demonstrated in Figure 6.2.

This continuum provides a useful model within which to analyse the processes of mentoring. It has the capacity to embrace the breadth

Outcome driven _____ Aspirational
needs   self-development

Figure 6.2 Mentoring focus continuum

and depth of mentoring activity, from one-to-one engagements to multimentoring processes. Thus it can be used as a diagnostic tool to assist in defining the parameters of mentoring relationships for individuals, and within organisations in the spirit of lifelong learning.

Conway (1998) suggests that mentoring is a powerful and effective organisational development strategy, as it preserves organisational wisdom, supports the development of leadership and smoothes the pathways of change. This contribution to both individual and organisational interests makes mentoring an appropriate and desirable activity within the context of 'a learning organisation' (Senge 1990, Hay 1995, Woodall & Winstanley 1998).

The NHS has launched the NHSU which makes explicit the NHS's belief in the value of the NHS as a learning organisation. It is intended to develop the NHSU as a corporate university in the future. The notion of a learning organisation also seems to be captured in the spirit of Clutterbuck & Megginson's *process model of mentoring* (1999, p. 22) (Fig. 6.3) and to fit with the continuum approach (Fig. 6.2).

The wider mentorship relationship

For the vast majority of the readers of this chapter, the mentorship processes and roles will not exist in an organisational vacuum. They will exist within the context of the organisation, and thus, in reality, the relationship may be tripartite, i.e. between the individual, the mentor and the organisational context (Fig. 6.4). However, it is useful to note that the contextual dimension may be transferable to other organisations in the sense that learning applied in one organisation can be used in another.

The emphasis on elements of the partnership is likely to fluctuate, and this depends on the desired outcomes of the relationship at any given time. The situation may be one of *maintenance mentorship*, or there may be a critical incident/event that might precipitate an intensive episode of working together. The incident may be rooted in the individual's immediate need, or in fact the need of the organisation – for example during merger activities when the organisation may require the individual to gain new skills and experiences either for a change of role or to seek alternative employment.

Active mentoring provides great benefits to the three partners:

- For the *individual*, it can offer a sounding board to develop ideas and new perspectives that can enhance job satisfaction, career prospects and help develop new networks.

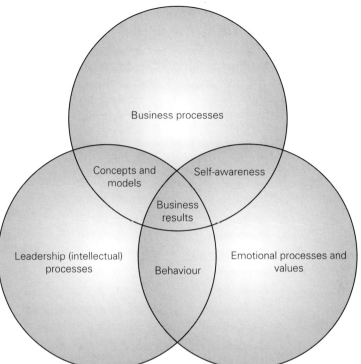

Figure 6.3 A process model (from Mentoring Executives and Directors by Clutterbuck & Megginson. Reprinted by permission of Elsevier Ltd)

- The *organisation* will benefit from more motivated staff and fresh ideas, and a reputation for valuing its staff and their contributions.
- The *mentor* too benefits by contributing to developing 'new talent' and has the opportunity to develop personal support skills,

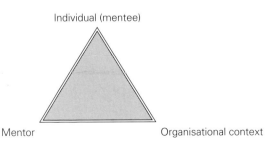

Figure 6.4 Three partners in mentorship relationships

169

Mentoring in the workplace

thus contributing to personal development. As the mentee, the mentor has the opportunity within the relationship to look at issues via a different perspective.

As mentorship is aimed at supporting the individual in developing self, both 'in the here and now' and for the future, a simple representation model is useful to see at a glance how the focus of the interaction might shift to meet the current need (Fig. 6.5).

Longer term relationship: ——————————————————— Strategic focus
(developmental/ facilitative)

Medium-term relationship: ——————————————————— More operationally driven
(support/supervisory, developmental) Minimally strategic

Short-term relationship: ——————————————————— Operationally driven
(supervisory, some developmental)

Figure 6.5 Focus of relationships

Characteristics of a mentor

Whilst it is fair to say that everyone can benefit from experiencing effective mentorship, the way the individual may wish to experience it will be different for many reasons.

Individual differences in personality, working environment, current role at work and other life responsibilities will all impact upon the context in which mentorship might best benefit each person.

However, the core characteristics of an effective mentor are consistent. The most important characteristics of all are a genuine willingness to be a mentor, and a genuine respect for the contribution and needs of others. Nevertheless, willingness and respect, however genuine, are not sufficient. Essential characteristics and skills include:

Managing self – making it work for you

- personal and professional integrity (there may be times when the mentee will wish to discuss issues of a confidential and sensitive nature)
- self-awareness and an ability to embrace ongoing personal development
- effective communication skills and an awareness of the impact of both verbal and non-verbal communication processes
- effective coaching skills
- effective listening skills (sometimes the individual mentee may find it difficult to be explicit)
- an ability to be non-directive (mentoring is *not* about telling the mentee what to do, nor is the mentor expected to have all the answers)
- being open to feedback
- being well organised, flexible, conscientious and committed to the process.

Responsibilities of the mentee

An effective mentorship relationship is one of equals and of partnerships. As the mentors are required to have responsibilities, the mentees too have responsibilities within the relationship, and the responsibility for managing the parameters of the relationship, particularly at the outset.

Mentees must be clear that the relationship is not one where it is expected that the mentor will take the lead in discussions. The prime beneficiary of the relationship is the *mentee*, who should be prepared to set the agenda. A short list of objectives to achieve for each meeting is a good way of staying focused. A good start is to either (in the case of the first meeting) give an overview of key issues, or (in the case of follow-up meetings) outline key points which have followed/been achieved since the last meeting. The mentee should always provide an up-to-date curriculum vitae as this will help the mentor to 'get a feel' for the experience of the mentee to date. This is particularly important if the relationship is new. Advice and suggestions about preparation of an appropriate curriculum vitae can be found in Chapter Nine.

Mentees are likely to be busy dealing with the pressures of work in the health care sector today, and the pressures of life in general. Thus one of the challenges is to know *how to set about determining what the mentee wants* from the mentorship relationship, and how that fits into the mentee's overall personal development framework.

Mentoring in the workplace

It is important that any one process in the continuum of personal and professional development activity is not seen in isolation from other activities. The model of self-development shown in Figure 6.6 (Hyde & Wright 1997) is a simple representation of how the mentor has a crucial role to play in the development of the individual; this model is also explicit in pointing to the personal responsibility of the mentee. However, if, as a result of working through this or a similar model, the mentee has a real *sticking point*, that may be an area where focused coaching from the mentor can help.

Choosing a mentor

You might like to think now, as part of your personal development activity, about how you will go about choosing a mentor. First of all, you need to think about the particular qualities and experiences you may want from the relationship. It may be that you already 'have your eye' on an individual. If that is so, you may find it useful to reflect on *why* you think this person will be a good mentor. It is likely that you have noticed, perhaps subconsciously, that the person you have in mind demonstrates certain traits or behaviours that you believe are worthy and/or effective. It is likely too that you will have felt *drawn* to the person – perhaps you cannot explain why – but unless you are going to feel comfortable with the person, an approach is not a good idea.

When you have identified a likely mentor, then you have to get in touch to see if this particular person is prepared to enter into a mentorship relationship. If you know the individual already, contact is easy. Choose your approach appropriately. If your potential mentor is not known to you personally (and therefore will not know you), it may be more appropriate to write, giving a very short overview of your experience and work context, and what you hope to achieve from the relationship in two or three concise bullet points. If you have worked through a personal development model (e.g. Fig. 6.6) this will give you more confidence and focus in choosing your objectives.

In the letter indicate that you will telephone in (for example) about 10 days' time to make the first appointment to *explore the potential of the relationship*. In the first instance a 30-minute time slot is sufficient to do that. This strategy gives the person an opportunity to 'say no' but also to see you without commitment. If the person refuses, do not take this personally – there may be a valid reason. This also gives you the opportunity to check out the person

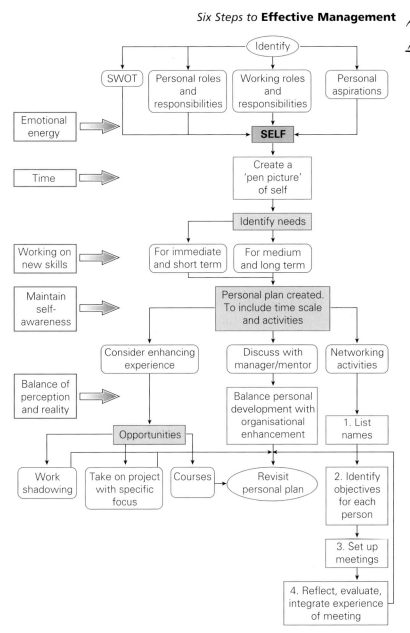

Figure 6.6 Self-development model reproduced fom Hyde & Wright 1997 with kind permission fom RCN Publishing Company

'face to face' in that context, and not to commit yourself before you have the opportunity to do that. If you have an introduction from a mutual colleague, all well and good, but do not be put off approaching the individual you have in mind if you do not have an introduction. A polite, structured approach is always acceptable, and even if your potential mentor is unable to enter into a relationship and declines your approach, you have lost nothing.

Meeting for the first time – exploring the potential of the relationship

This is where you present yourself as a competent professional person. You must arrive promptly, dress appropriately (different industries have different dress codes) and be prepared to take the lead in the meeting, using the objectives you have prepared earlier! You will need to be clear about the parameters of the potential relationship, and the (approximate) number of times a year you hope to meet. Often in a mentorship relationship which is not a 'professional (clinical) supervision' one, once or twice a year will be enough. Remember that the first interview is two sided: the potential mentor has to agree, and you have to feel comfortable and psychologically safe. If you do not, it is no good progressing with the relationship. That is why it is important that the first appointment is one to *explore potential*, rather than to seal the knot! If it works for both of you, you can go ahead and make the next appointment. If you are unsure, do not commit yourself. If the relationship does not go ahead, it is courteous to write a short 'thank you' letter in acknowledgement of the time spent with you.

Focused mentoring – mentoring underperforming staff

Chapter Four examines the broad issues of performance management, and clearly in a generalist textbook such as this is it not appropriate (or possible) to examine performance management in detail. Readers who have a special interest should refer to specialist texts such as Armstrong (2000). Nevertheless the basic processes which are contained in the mentoring relationship are those that can be used in a more focused way to help staff develop new and current skills, and thus improve their overall performance. It is likely that the mentor in these circumstances will be an individual who is working in the same organisation as the mentee, although that is not always the case – it depends very much on the role the mentee has, and how this role needs developing. However, what is mandatory is that the relationship is entered into in a spirit of development and cooperation, rather than one of 'improve, or else'.

The reader should have the confidence to adapt core skills to different contexts, and this is done by 'working backwards', i.e. identifying what the key outcomes of the process are to be. This will enable the relationship to focus on the priority actions.

Once these priorities have been agreed by all parties then the process can begin. Note that this is an instance when the tripartite relationship (see Fig. 6.4) is explicit. If the individual is not performing optimally, this impacts on the organisation, and thus the organisation may require and support an active, focused mentorship arrangement.

A simple 'helping' model, such the one adapted from Egan's 'EUA model' (Egan 2002) outlined in Table 6.2, may be useful in establishing a working relationship when the explicit outcome is one of developing the performance of an individual to meet specific objectives. ('EUA' in Egan's work refers to the processes of *exploration, understanding* and *action*, and can easily be adapted to fit a mentoring relationship, or in fact a relationship of clinical/professional supervision.)

Egan originally devised his model as one to be used in a professional counselling relationship. An important point for the reader to note is the *transferability* of concepts and processes. Any communication relationship between two (or more) people must have some core themes. These will be applied and interpreted in different ways according to the agenda, context and required outcomes of the communication relationship.

Similar processes are apparent in textbooks on leadership, change management, communication and a range of other disciplines. These disciplines may have their own *language* for the processes and the relationship, but the basic core activities remain the same. This to some extent explains the confusion between terminology and definitions of processes, relationships and activities.

In a learning organisation, the ability to use skills in different contexts and in different ways is a useful resource for any individual, either manager or clinician.

A learning organisation should see the development of underperforming staff as a positive professional development activity, and not one of punitive blame and finger pointing. Clinical governance makes this very clear. Reducing the blame culture is seen as a key factor in developing a high quality service. The relationship between effective leadership and change management processes

Mentoring in the workplace

Managing self – making it work for you

Table 6.2 Mentorship for performance development (based on Egan 2002)

Exploration	Understanding	Action
What are the issues?	Discuss and 'unpick' issues	Set timescale – usually staged
What do we want/need to achieve and what are the priorities?	Analyse factors – tools such as SWOT analysis may be useful in identifying key factors and their relationships with the mentee	Prioritise actions and identify any resources (e.g. time)
Who are the stakeholders?	Seek understanding of factors in context, including the agenda of various stakeholders	Identify key stakeholders
What are the parameters of the mentor/ mentee relationship?	Seek understanding about what each can bring to the relationship and establish ground rules	Identify a means of evaluation, which then feeds back into 'exploration'
Set 'ground rules' for confidentiality etc.	Devise a strategy	Prepare an outline plan

(although the term mentorship is not used, the processes are referred to implicitly) and their contribution to quality within a framework of clinical governance is made explicit by Scally & Donaldson (1998).

Without a collection of individuals who have the basic skills of mentorship, helping or supervision, an organisation will have difficulty in becoming truly a *learning organisation*.

Cultural change is slow, and managing change (see Chapter Three) is a challenge. Stoter (1997) emphasises that good staff support is an indication of the value the organisation places on staff. The application of effective mentorship principles as part of the organisation's acknowledgement of the importance of people as its greatest asset can play an important part in personal and professional development, so ultimately the quality of the service is enhanced. Mentorship is not a luxury or a management fad. It is a real tool for quality, and an important element in achieving a healthy learning organisation.

Discussion questions

- Outline the key activities that make up the mentorship role.
- What are the characteristics of an effective mentor?
- What are the benefits of mentorship to (a) the mentor and (b) the person being mentored?
- How can the mentoring process contribute to the quality of service delivery and the achievement of the organisation's business objectives?

References

Armstrong M 2000 Strategic human resource management – a guide to action. Kogan Page, London

Clutterbuck D, Megginson D 1999 Mentoring executives and directors. Butterworth-Heinemann, Oxford

Conway C 1998 Strategies for mentoring – a blueprint for successful organisational development. John Wiley, Chichester

Department of Health 1997 The new NHS: modern, dependable. Department of Health, London

Department of Health 1998a A first class service – quality in the new NHS. Department of Health, London

Department of Health 1998b Working together: securing a quality workforce for the NHS. Department of Health, London

Department of Health 2000 The NHS plan: a plan for investment, a plan for reform. Department of Health, London

Department of Health 2001a Shifting the balance of power in the NHS. Department of Health, London

Department of Health 2001b The Bristol Inquiry (The Kennedy Report). Department of Health, London

Egan G 2002 The skilled helper, 7th edn. Brooks/Cole, Australia

Gibb S 2002 Learning and development – processes, practices and perspectives at work. Palgrave Macmillan, Basingstoke

Hay J 1995 Transformational mentoring – creating development alliances for changing organisational cultures. (2nd edition published 1999.) Sherwood Publishing, Watford

Hyde J 1988a Lean on me. Nursing Standard 22: 24

Hyde J 1988b A guide to the role of the mentor. Royal College of Nursing, London

Mentoring in the workplace

Hyde J, Wright A 1997 Self development. Nursing Management 4(3): 10–11

Scally G, Donaldson L J 1998 Clinical governance and the drive for quality improvement in the new NHS in England. British Medical Journal 317: 61–65

Senge P M 1990 The fifth discipline – the art and practice of the learning organization. Century Business, London

Stoter D J 1997 Staff support in health care. Blackwell Science, Oxford

Whittaker M, Cartwright A 2000 The mentoring manual. Gower, Aldershot

Woodall J, Winstanley D 1998 Management development – strategy and practice. Blackwell Business, Oxford

Application **6:1**

Carol Marrow

Engaging in clinical supervision:

nurses' perspectives from focus group discussions

In this application, Marrow presents a short overview of some findings from her research into clinical supervision. As Hyde mentions in Chapter Six, the terms mentorship and clinical supervision are not synonymous, yet the processes involved are similar; it is the context and focus taken that are often different. Clinical supervision as you would expect is grounded specifically in clinical practice, whilst mentorship embraces a broader remit. Nevertheless, the skills in one process are transferable to the other. Note also that clinical supervision, like mentorship, can be delivered either in a one-to-one relationship or within a group.

INTRODUCTION

Supporting nurses in clinical practice is important for both their personal and professional development and the resulting quality of patient care (Butterworth et al 1998, Marrow & Yaseen 1998, Marrow 2000). Further developing knowledge and critical appraisal skills in communities of practice helps to promote clinical effectiveness (Kitson et al 1996), thus underpinning the principles of clinical governance. The role of clinical supervision was the focus of the research project (Marrow 2000) outlined in this application which illustrates some of the processes and outcomes of a collaborative action research study that explored clinical supervision for nurses.

Project findings

The findings from this research project illustrate that through the supportive, dynamic process of clinical supervision, nurses engaging in communities of practice developed reflexivity, self and professional awareness and enhanced patient care skills.

To enable the supervisory process to be more effective, the participants were encouraged to reflect on practice by using a diary. Although the diaries were not utilised explicitly for collecting research data, they enhanced the research process by allowing a more rigorous recording of practice issues to take place. The issues identified were then fed into the subsequent focus group discussions.

The findings from the research were positive in terms of the process and outcomes of clinical supervision. The data highlight that the participants felt substantially supported in their role through the impact of clinical supervision. Moreover, they perceived clinical supervision as helping to increase their knowledge, questioning abilities, reflective skills and competence.

The data from the focus group discussions highlighted tangible benefits for clinical practice. These included changes in care protocols, the development of new care protocols and improved relationships with patients. However, constraints around the successful implementation of clinical supervision were also noted and main concerns focused on lack of support and quality time.

A brief overview of key themes that emerged is presented here.

PROFESSIONAL SUPPORT

The participants overwhelmingly found a great deal of support from linking with other practitioners.

- 'I've found it really supportive because I have been so isolated and I'm sure XXX feels the same way because we are the only two at this end ... . It is very rare that we actually get to be together. So to have another two people doing the same job, I find it really supportive. It's been good.'
- 'I remember saying before we got into groups, Oh roll on clinical supervision. I felt desperately in need of that ... the fact that I have had to change and the concerns that I had from being a single-handed practitioner to having staff members. I feel that the group helps me.'

A number of other studies supports the view that clinical supervision is valuable in helping practitioners. Scanlon & Weir (1997), for example, investigated the perceptions and experiences of clinical supervision for ten mental health nurses and found that they felt supported and valued by their supervisors and that the supervision helped to safeguard the intensity of the nurse/patient relationship. Swain (1995) importantly suggests that nurses need to be able to help themselves (perhaps in the form of clinical supervision) before they can help others.

CHANGES IN PRACTICE

There were numerous discussions that linked changes in clinical practice with clinical supervision. Some participants reported that as a result of the clinical supervision process, new improved protocols had been introduced. This is exciting as it suggests tangible evidence of the importance of clinical supervision for quality patient care.

- 'There has been a specific change in my clinical area (gynaecology). There was a patient who I felt I had failed in some way. The ward protocol offered the patient a type of care (to look after her baby that was resident with her on the ward) but I was unable to do this at this particular time. I discussed it with my supervisor in the clinical supervision session and we changed the protocol.'
- 'My approach in the way I approach the patients is developing. I can see them more as a whole, more so than I used to. Through the discussions we have had in clinical supervision ... she makes me see different aspects that I have taken to my dealings with my patients that I probably didn't see before.'

There is not much literature on clinical supervision that identifies improvements in clinical and patient care. However, through a case study, Johns (1993) describes how through the use of reflection and supervision a nurse practitioner was able to untangle the complexities of caring and develop more therapeutic relationships. Marrow & Yaseen's (1998) study highlighted positive changes in clinical management and care protocols.

PROBLEMS IN CLINICAL SUPERVISION

Management issues

Many of the participants felt that management did not always support either the implementation and/or the outcomes of clinical supervision. However, there was a number of constraints at the time of the preparation and execution of this project. Other priorities, particularly the trust mergers, were taking up most of the manager's time.

- 'I took some issues from clinical supervision to management and met with a negative response, so I have brought it to the focus group. There are networks available that management could use to inform relevant bodies that there is a problem in this particular area, we were not happy about the response.'

Finding time for clinical supervision

It is apparent that new initiatives such as clinical supervision involve much practitioner commitment and energy. Support from everyone is

Engaging in clinical supervision: nurses' perspectives

181

therefore essential to maintain the momentum. Finding the time to carry out clinical supervision was a big issue in this study; many of the participants had to engage in clinical supervision in their own time or by telephone.

- 'The problem with the staff and the way we work now is you just don't have the time and energy to talk about practice. This is why you have to have such a commitment for these sessions. You really have to think hard about it and sometimes the pressure is on you to keep it going. I have to plan my session at least the night before. So we are taking a lot of our own time doing it ... .'

Shortage of time emerged as a key feature. Many practitioners perceive clinical supervision as an extra chore rather than an implicit part of everyday practice. Thus the realistic amount of time required for regular clinical supervision needs consideration if it is to be integrated into the working day.

REFLECTIONS ON THE PROCESS

Effective clinical supervision is aimed at supporting and empowering practitioners engaged in communities of practice. Evidence from this study highlights that as a result of the reflective process of clinical supervision, a number of the participants felt more motivated, knowledgeable, competent, empowered and less stressed. They also promoted leadership and care initiatives in their work environments, thus emphasising the importance of supportive strategies and effective leadership in developing nurses and thus the quality of care.

Difficulties are frequently experienced when implementing new initiatives like clinical supervision. Many problems were identified in this study, not least finding the quality time for entering into clinical supervision. Employers need to give commitment to clinical supervision, and practitioners need to perceive it as beneficial for their personal and professional development and therefore incorporate the concept into their working practice rather than see it as an extra chore. In today's challenging health sector, support is essential to ensure practitioners are developed to their full potential.

Those who have experienced effective clinical supervision report they would be reluctant to imagine life without it!

References

Butterworth T, Faugier J, Burnard P (eds) 1998 Clinical supervision and mentorship in nursing, 2nd edn. Stanley Thornes, Cheltenham

Johns C 1993 Guided reflection. In: Palmer A, Burns S, Bulman C (eds) Reflective practice in nursing: the growth of the professional practitioner. Blackwell, London

Kitson A, Ahmed L B, Harvey G, Seers K, Thompson D R 1996 From research to practice: one organisational model for promoting research-based practice. Journal of Advanced Nursing 23: 430–440

Marrow C E 2000 Supervision on line (SOL): an evaluation of video conferencing technology as a medium for clinical supervision in nursing. Research report. St Martin's College, Lancaster

Marrow C E, Yaseen T 1998 Developing supervision in adult/general nursing. In: Butterworth T, Faugier J, Burnard P (eds) Clinical supervision and mentorship in nursing, 2nd edn. Stanley Thornes, Cheltenham, Chapter 7

Scanlon C, Weir W S 1997 Learning from practice? Mental health nurses' perceptions and experiences of clinical supervision. Journal of Advanced Nursing 26(2): 295–303

Swain G 1995 Clinical supervision: the principles and process. Community Practitioners and Health Visitors Association, London

Engaging in clinical supervision: nurses' perspectives

Application **6:2**

Kate Jagger

Providing mentorship and supervision

In this application Jagger discusses the role of the mentor in an educational context, and includes some comments taken from individuals experiencing the mentorship relationship. Note how positive a good relationship can be, but that an ineffective relationship can produce negative experiences. This is true in any context.

INTRODUCTION

This application gives some examples of effective mentorship at work in an educational context. The following criteria are important to ensure a successful experience:

- Mentors need to have a supportive, facilitatory style.
- Mentorship requires negotiated dedicated time.
- Mentorship should be formed with a clear contract of how it will work.
- Mentorship requires a commitment to achieve agreed objectives.
- Mentors require preparation for their role.
- Mutual respect in the relationship is essential.

CHOOSING A MENTOR

Choosing the right mentor is critical to success. Often, the first experience of mentorship is one to support learning during an educational course. This relationship is focused upon achieving a successful outcome, yet the processes are transferable to any individual workplace as a formal way of evaluating performance and supporting ongoing development.

Where mentorship, preceptorship, clinical supervision and other helping relationships are part of an organisation's culture, or part of an education structure, there is no doubt of their potency and impact in enabling staff to feel supported and empowered.

The following comments are taken from a group of 70 qualified staff undertaking educational programmes where mentorship is a key element of delivery. The participants chose their own mentors, and workshops for mentors were carried out at various stages during the 6 month duration of the courses.

REFLECTING ON MENTORSHIP

Below are some examples of how people describe their experience of mentorship in an educational context.

Staff nurse in an acute hospital setting
● 'XXX has been very helpful and supportive throughout the course. I have nothing but praise for her help.'

Interestingly, the nurse does not attempt to analyse the mentor's role here, but the important thing for her is that she felt supported, and was enabled to move through the programme successfully.

Deputy manager of a resource centre within the social services
● 'I have experienced a high level of support and supervision from my mentor. We have had regular discussions on many subjects including joint working, assessment, care plans and my proposed project. We have usually met on a weekly basis and sometimes more regularly if I need to.'

This relationship is defined as mentorship by the person receiving the support, and that may surprise some readers who may feel that the description of the relationship is what is known as 'clinical supervision'. However, this does not matter; what is important is the *quality* of the relationship and its effectiveness in terms of outcomes.

Head occupational therapist in an acute hospital setting
● 'Excellent support and guidance – we met once a month plus a number of telephone calls. We discussed my progress towards meeting my objectives and my progress and feelings about the course. She has also helped by constantly monitoring my work type and load.'

Staff nurse in a community hospital
● 'Excellent support from my mentor who was enthusiastic throughout. I had unlimited time for discussion around all the subjects related to the course. My work was read and discussed at different stages throughout, and on the final completion.'

Providing mentorship and supervision

Six Steps to **Effective Management**

Ward sister in an acute hospital

- 'My mentor (XXX) was a mainstay especially in the beginning of the programme when I needed to see her the most. She was always constructive in her feedback.'

Health visitor in a medical practice

- 'My mentor was excellent, she was supportive without being rigid, directive or intrusive. She was always available.'

Staff nurse in a community mental health unit where supervision is part of the organisation's culture

- 'I have had excellent support from my mentor/supervisor. We meet on a monthly basis, for formal discussions, and informal discussions on a weekly basis. We explore the formulation and development of carers' assessments.'

Senior clinical nurses in an acute hospital

- 'Through working with my mentor and having the opportunity to explore professional and personal issues I have gained in confidence.'
- 'I would like to have had more time with my mentor – with the pressure of work it was difficult for both of us to meet regularly – however it did give the opportunity to discuss issues arising from the workshops at a more personal and in depth level. I feel the support during those sessions compensated for the lack of time we spent together.'

MAKE SURE YOU MAKE TIME

Mentorship is time consuming. Anyone who is considering entering into a relationship either as a mentor or as a mentee must think about the issue seriously.

The following feedback demonstrates a lack of partnership and focus between the mentor and mentee when making agreements about expectations and commitment of both parties. Agreeing the parameter of the contract in mentorship, preceptorship and supervision is imperative to the success of the relationship, be it a short- or long-term one.

Staff nurses in an acute hospital

- 'No reflection at all on my mentor – she gave me as much time and attention as she could. She had constraints of taking up a new post in a very stressful and busy environment.'
- 'I realise that the pressure of work all round makes such meetings difficult to arrange which can be frustrating.'

Senior clinical nurse in an acute hospital

- 'The difficulties are when a person chooses the wrong mentor ... if they do not have the confidence to be up front about this with that person. I have to admit I have not met with my mentor after our first initial meeting, as she was for me undoubtedly the wrong choice.'

Staff nurse in a community setting

- 'Little direct support from my mentor. It was up to me to contact her including travelling. It was difficult to work together, but on the occasions we did I felt more effort on her part was needed.'

CONCLUSION

All the above comments were made from the perspective of an educational mentorship relationship, but the principles may emerge in any context. An effective relationship is a positive experience for both parties, but a negative one can have a long-lasting impact. Make sure you can give commitment to it.

Providing mentorship and supervision

Chapter **Seven**

Managing self:

lifestyle and wellbeing

Nick Hyde

- A balanced lifestyle
- Physical and psychological fitness
- Maintaining a healthy self
- SMART goal setting

- Exercise – stamina/strength/suppleness
- Rest and relaxation
- Diet
- A positive environment

OVERVIEW

This chapter focuses on you, the reader. In the busy melee of professional life, too often we ignore our own needs because every bit of our time is focused on work. A healthy balance between self-wellbeing, personal life and professional life is important so that you can give your best in every sphere of your life.

Here, Hyde gives an overview of the process of goal setting to achieve balance in your lifestyle, and stresses the importance of looking after yourself in a sensible way. He offers a strategy to help you achieve this goal.

INTRODUCTION

Many books and magazines are published every year highlighting the benefits of physical fitness and diet, the covers awash with fine physical specimens. Furthermore, each month a new diet and exercise regimen is endorsed by a celebrity, claiming miraculous intervention. Unfortunately this is not reality, as time spent at work fails to allow sufficient time to read the magazine, let alone follow its advice. This chapter will reinforce the focus on *self* and how to manage your body within the dynamic world of leadership.

WHY LOOK AFTER SELF?

As a professional, people will look to you for inspiration. Furthermore, they expect of you a certain bearing, charisma, knowledge and presence. To achieve this, you need to be fit and well. However, this does not mean that you must be the replica of an Olympian or a professional sportsman. Far from it; fitness must be taken in context, for an injured athlete whilst unfit, is however by general description, very fit. In business, a leader must be 'fit for purpose' and the day-to-day stresses of life, which means not only being physically fit, but psychologically fit too. A balanced lifestyle can help you achieve this.

Physical fitness

Countless research articles have highlighted the benefits of physical fitness; some benefits are outlined below:

- reduced levels of obesity
- reduced risk of coronary heart disease
- healthier into old age
- general improvements in health.

Psychological fitness

The greater the level of physical fitness, the greater the benefits to psychological fitness. Benefits to psychological fitness include:

- greater self-confidence
- higher levels of concentration

Managing self: lifestyle and wellbeing

- improved self-awareness
- increased levels of intrinsic motivation.

Although the above points are not exhaustive, it is easy for leaders to recognise and apply these benefits to self and to leadership performance.

Many find the imperative to keep fit daunting as keeping fit is not just about attending the gym – it is about maintaining an appropriate and realistic lifestyle.

MAINTAINING A HEALTHY SELF THROUGH LIFESTYLE

By focusing on four components of lifestyle and outlining a simple psychological skill, you can begin to take positive steps to achieve and maintain a healthy lifestyle.

SMART goal setting for self

The theory of goal setting is well established as a motivational tool and provides a useful approach to setting lifestyle targets. By planning and setting realistic goals around your objectives, your attention can be focused on the task to be achieved. Having done that, the next step is to develop strategies for achieving those goals.

Planning to be SMART

By using the acronym SMART (specific, measurable, achievable, realistic, time related) you can begin to plan, for example: *Goal* – to set aside time for exercise that I enjoy.

- *Specific* – Specific goal setting tends to be more effective than setting subjective goals. The goal is fairly specific as it focuses on an enjoyable exercise, in this case we'll say swimming. 'I must set time aside for swimming' is the specific goal.
- *Measurable* – By adding a further statement, the initial goal becomes more measurable: 'I will set aside 2 hours for swimming per week, by going to the pool for 30 minutes four times a week.'
- *Achievable* – The goal has to be achievable, as there must be the flexibility to modify goals as result of sickness or extreme business commitment. Failure to do this results in a feeling of failure or demotivation, as, in reality, circumstances do change.

Managing self – making it work for you

For example, in times of unprecedented business pressures (such as an urgent project) the new goal might read: 'I will put aside two 30-minute swimming sessions a week until a week on Monday when the project has finished.'

- *Realistic* – Do not bite off more than you can chew, particularly in relation to the amount of exercise you are planning, if the goal represents a significant lifestyle change. To set a goal of swimming every day may be unrealistic. Goals must be challenging, but not out of sight. If on Monday, the meeting runs over into your swimming time you have failed on the first day of the week! This will cause you to feel demotivated, and that you have failed in your goal.

- *Time related* – Try to ensure that there is a realistic time-related aspect, so that you do not put off the goal.

You must be committed to accepting the set goals. You may consider drawing up a strategy or mission statement to help focus your mind and achieve your goal.

Lifestyle components

Exercise

The importance of exercise and its effect on physical fitness are well documented, but what does this mean to you? In the first instance by focusing on stamina, strength and suppleness, significant lifestyle benefits will be realised.

- *Stamina* – Increasing the number of times per week you are out of breath will increase your stamina as well as having positive effects upon your heart and lungs (check of course with your doctor before embarking upon serious exercise). It may be you walk up the stairs in the office every morning rather than taking the lift, you may choose to get off the bus or train a stop earlier and walk home or to the office.

- *Strength* – Increasing strength by weight bearing will have many health benefits and particularly into middle and old age as this helps to ensure that muscle mass and bone density are maintained. It is now common for many of us to go to the gym or attend exercise classes; however, carrying the shopping home from the supermarket is strength training.

- *Suppleness* – Simply by putting your joints through a full range of movement and a gentle system of stretching will enhance your sense of wellbeing. Reaching up above your head whilst standing on tiptoes will gently stretch many major muscle groups and help ensure your structural health.

The suggestions outlined above are basic and easy to do, but will make a different to those in the most sedentary occupations. Remember that exercise should be fun and thus can provide an excellent source of relaxation.

Rest and relaxation

Both rest and relaxation must play a large part in the professional's weekly diary. Time away from stressful projects or just day-to-day work is vital in order to recharge the batteries. This time is perhaps spent with family or participating in a hobby that you enjoy. Likewise adequate rest allows the body and mind to recover – this should mean between 6 and 8 hours of sleep per night.

Diet

In an age obsessed with image, diet has become a term used to create such an image. The countless number of diets on the market make the trip to the supermarket seem like a minefield. However, it need not be the case. By sticking to the basic principle of eating a balanced diet containing a combination of carbohydrate (60%), fat (25%) and protein (15%) with necessary minerals and vitamins coming from vegetables in the diet, healthy eating is ensured. It is important to manage portion size. If you eat more than you burn, however 'well balanced' the diet, you will increase fat storage and thus put on weight.

Also included under the heading of a balanced diet is your hydration level. It is critically important that the body is well hydrated in order to maintain good health. Drinking about 2 litres of water-based fluid per day will ensure that you are adequately hydrated. However, this does not include alcohol, tea and coffee, as they will remove fluid from the body as a result of their diuretic effect.

Creating a positive environment

As a professional, you are often more concerned for your charges than for yourself. However, it is critical that your working environment is not only safe, but also well ventilated and has as much natural light as is possible.

The benefits ...

Many professionals will cite the lack of time as an excuse to explain the lack of a healthy lifestyle. However, with a small amount of time management and organisation, an effective outcome can be achieved.

CONCLUSION

It must be stressed that this outline is not a stand-alone regimen, but merely a toolbox to give the individual pointers and suggestions to help maintain a healthier self.

Positive wellbeing may be the missing piece to your professional jigsaw. Why not repay the investment in your career with some investment in self?

Discussion questions

- What elements of your lifestyle contribute directly to your wellbeing?
- What are the benefits of a balanced lifestyle?

Managing self: lifestyle and wellbeing

Chapter **Eight**

Managing stress for yourself

Michael J Cook

- The definition of stress
- Levels of stress
- The job strain model

- Environmental stressors
- Coping with stress

OVERVIEW

In this chapter Cook gives an overview of some theoretical views of stress and, in emphasising that stress is a normal factor in our working lives, suggests a positive approach to cope with it.

INTRODUCTION

Stress is an overused and abused word used to describe anything from pressure as a result of a delayed train, to overwhelming disorders such as post traumatic stress syndrome. More often than not, the experience of stress is perceived to have negative impact.

Stress is defined as 'a physical, mental, psychological or spiritual response to a stressor' (Narasi 1994, p. 73). A stressor is defined as an experience in a person's environment that is evaluated by a person as being taxing or exceeding resources and threatening the sense of wellbeing (Lazarus & Folkman 1984). In other words, stress is a series of events. It is important too to bear in mind that what might stress one individual might not be of any consequence

Managing self – making it work for you

to another. There are many variables which impact on how a stressor is perceived, particularly the context in which it occurs, and the individual's previous experiences.

LEVELS OF STRESS

When something happens to us which we interpret as a stressor, we respond and make a series of judgements: is this event potentially harmful to us or people we care about or are responsible for? Can we cope with the consequences of the events? The answers we give determine the level of stress we experience. Several factors interact to determine the stress levels experienced. These include the demands made on the person and particularly the autonomy or degree of control people have over the issues. Payne (1979), looking at this factor in the work situation, considered occupational stress to be a function of the interaction between demands, supports and constraints at work. Payne suggested that support is an important factor in reducing work stress as it can help to neutralise the demands and stress experienced.

THE JOB STRAIN MODEL

Karasek (1979) developed a job strain model (Fig. 8.1). This addresses levels of staff satisfaction with the amount of decision, authority and task discretion they have over their work. It is suggested that staff whose jobs are characterised by high demands and

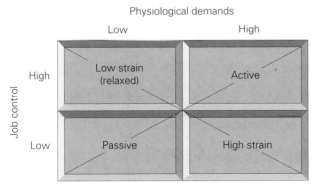

Figure 8.1 Job strain model (reproduced with kind permission from Karasek 1979, © Administrative Science Quarterly)

low decision latitude (control) are at greater risk of poor psychological wellbeing. According to this model, two dimensions – job demands and decision latitude (job control) – make it possible to distinguish between four main job types:

- *High strain* – high demands and low decision latitude
- *Low strain* – ('relaxed') jobs; low demands and high decision latitude
- *Active* – high demands and high decision latitude
- *Passive* – low demands and low decision latitude.

The model suggests that the lowest levels of psychological wellbeing and the highest levels of symptoms and diseases are to be found in the high strain group. Another important factor from Karasek's work is that people in active jobs seem to have more potential to access learning and personal development, as well as to actively participate in social life, than those people in passive jobs. Which job is best for the individual depends on what they are seeking. A person looking for personal development and learning as priority should perhaps look for an active job whilst a relaxed job is preferable for people who seek to ensure psychological wellbeing and good health.

ENVIRONMENTAL STRESSORS

The cumulative effect of chronic daily pressure is an important cause of stress. Williams et al (1998) identify the following specific environmental stressors that nurses face:

- unpredictable staffing and scheduling
- lack of role clarity
- low involvement in decision making
- poor status
- poor support.

You might like to reflect on your own feelings with respect to each of these factors. Are any of these issues important in your working environment? If so, what can you do about them?

COPING WITH STRESS

It is important to acknowledge that each of the bullet points has a personal context and a wider, less personal context. Covey (1989) refers to circles of concern and circles of influence. He refers to the importance of dealing with the areas of circles of concern and expending less energy on the circles of influence. In other words, deal with issues that you can deal with directly in each of the bullet points and be less concerned with the areas that are not under your direct control. By dealing with direct areas it is possible in the longer term to exert pressure over the areas of influence.

Bennett et al (1999) identify three areas on which to focus with respect to stress. These are:

- environmental factors, such as working conditions and working practices
- developing individual skills to function well and with confidence
- stress management skills for those who need them.

A study undertaken by Quinn (1998) within a NHS Trust identified that:

> Giving employees more variety in tasks and more participation in decision making may decrease the risk of psychological ill health and sickness absence. Improving support structures may have the same effect. It may not be possible to decrease the demands of the job, but stress is not an inevitable consequence if greater support and job control are provided.

CONCLUSION

The issues discussed above have identified that for health care provision to improve staff must be aware of the stress factors in their workplace. Only then can staff identify their reactions to these stress factors and consider options for dealing with them. One thing for sure – stress is here to stay – we need to learn how to deal with it effectively.

Discussion questions

- What support mechanisms do you employ or encourage for yourself or staff? Could these be improved?
- In the areas where you do well, which points warrant celebration?

Managing stress for yourself

Six Steps to **Effective Management**

References

Bennett P, Scott L, Harling K 1999 Stress busters. Nursing Times 95(50): 28–29

Covey S 1989 The seven habits of highly effective people. Simon and Schuster, London

Karasek R A 1979 Job demands, job decision latitude and mental strain: implications for job redesign. Administrative Science Quarterly 24: 285–308

Lazarus R, Folkman S 1984 Stress appraisal and coping. Springer, New York

Narasi B 1994 A tool for living through stress. Nursing Management 25(9): 73–75

Payne R 1979 Demands, supports, constraints and psychological health. In: McKay C, Cox T (eds) Response to stress: occupational aspects. IPC Business Press, London

Quinn L 1998 effects of stress in an NHS trust: a study. Nursing Standard 13(3): 36–41

Williams S, Michie S, Pattani S 1998 Improving the health of the workforce. Report on the partnership on the health of the NHS workforce. Nuffield Trust, London

Managing self – making it work for you

Chapter **Nine**

Enhancing and developing your career via your curriculum vitae, personal development planning and networking

Julie Hyde

- Types of CV
- Creating a structured CV
- Career breaks
- Personal development planning
- Networking

O V E R V I E W

Selling yourself is an important part of professional life. A good, focused curriculum vitae is the 'shop window' onto you and your career achievement. It is this document that will get you an interview for a job. Here Hyde points out some key points to remember when preparing your CV, and outlines the process of professional networking.

INTRODUCTION

Over the past decade, the pattern of work for everyone within and outside the health care sector has changed. As structures have been flattened and management responsibility pushed further down the hierarchy, we have seen fewer posts which give one the opportunity to 'try out' the job. Gone are the 'support posts', gone are many middle management posts, and the end result is that the more senior you become, the fewer posts there are. Writers have described 'a career climbing frame' rather than 'a career ladder'. This implies that an individual may make lateral career moves, as well as career steps 'up the ladder'. Paradoxically, whilst this has been happening in non-clinical posts in the NHS (as well as in managerial roles outside the health care industry), the introduction of the nurse grading system, along with the move towards specialism as opposed to generalism (as in the medical career model), tended to confound this pattern. Nurses were discouraged from taking sideways moves into another specialty once they were beyond a D grade, as this would 'dilute' their specialty expertise on which the grade promotion system depended. Whilst for the organisation this is a legitimate way of managing scarce resources, for many individual nurses who wished to stay in clinical posts, this felt like a barrier to progression. The recent introduction of 'nurse consultant' posts and the recommendations of *Agenda for Change* (DoH 2003) aim to address this concern.

The introduction of formal human resource practices into the NHS does mean that formal job application processes are now well established. Gone are the days (for nurses) when a little chat with matron would suffice! Thus, from day one, we need to be developing the skills and tools to 'sell' ourselves in the marketplace, as the exciting concept of portfolio careers gains ground.

Apart from the obvious things, like being able to do the job and holding the relevant licence to practise, there are a number of 'career skills' to collect in your personal development toolbox. Three of the key skills are:

- the ability to produce a focused and 'living' curriculum vitae (CV)
- proactive personal development planning via your personal development plan (PDP)
- structured networking.

Managing self – making it work for you

PREPARING YOUR CURRICULUM VITAE

An up-to-date curriculum vitae (CV) is an important tool for us all. It serves three purposes:

- it acts as a focal point to assist you to capture your skills, knowledge and achievements
- it serves as a basis for your PDP and thus is likely to inform your appraisal process at work
- it acts as a marketing tool to 'sell' you when you are seeking new opportunities, whether that is a particular new job, or if you are just testing the market.

The preparation of this important document follows a number of stages. Bear in mind however that for most people one CV is not enough. That is not to say that your CV represents someone other than yourself – quite the reverse. Your CV gives you the opportunity to add emphasis to your experience and to show the transferability of your knowledge and skills in the workplace. Clearly, a number of circumstances unique to you will inform your CV and CV preparation. If you qualified last week, and you entered your career straight from school, you will have less material to include in your CV than someone who has been in the profession for some 20 years or more. But the important fact to bear in mind is that the *principles* and *processes* involved in crafting a CV are the same. Your CV is not a fixed document; it is one that grows and develops and evolves with *your* growth, development and evolution.

An effective CV puts the right emphasis upon your experience, and clearly, that emphasis is informed and shaped by the purpose for which you are preparing it. As a means of illustrating this, we will assume that one individual (let's call this person Chris) might want to have three current CVs. CV1 will be a baseline, a collection of information capturing the uniqueness of Chris as a professional and as a person.

Subsequent CVs will take the same material as in CV1 and address the emphasis to match the purpose. If Chris were applying for a job in a clinical setting, then the emphasis in CV2 would be on clinical experience. Even then there could be two ways of dealing with this clinical experience. If Chris were applying for a job requiring very specialised clinical expertise, for example, that of a clinical nurse specialist in renal nursing, CV2 would need to have a detailed clinical focus. If, however, the role/job Chris was applying for required a more general focus, then Chris's skills would need to

201

be packaged in a different way. There would not be so much emphasis on the clinical expertise in renal nursing, rather Chris would generalise past clinical experience to a broader perspective, for example to facilitate management of a medical unit. Chris would not be expected to be an expert in all the specialties represented in the medical unit, but would draw on overall experience to manage the unit as a whole.

Chris would need to make a judgement about the culture and values of the organisation/unit. An aggressively business oriented organisation may want to see different things emphasised in a CV than a charity funded organisation.

All CVs will include the individual's professional and educational qualifications, as well as professional and personal experiences. In the two hypothetical scenarios above (i.e. renal nursing and medical unit), it is more likely that Chris's clinical/management experience will be the crucial focus.

However, if Chris were applying for a job in an academic establishment, CV3 will need to include much greater detail about the types and levels of academic courses, and include in detail any publications, conference papers, etc. This is not to say that these are not of interest in CV1 and CV2, but it is a matter of emphasis. If Chris were applying for a job in a sharp business culture, to emphasise the number and range of academic courses achieved might cause the manager looking at the CV to worry that Chris is more interested in doing courses than getting the job done. It is all a matter of organisational culture and inherent core values.

Conversely, the organisational culture of an academic establishment values as currency the academic processes and achievements that the applicant can offer, and thus these must be given in detail. A word of warning here though – the level of detail must be offered on a sliding scale, from present times, backwards. A 2-hour in-house course completed some 20 years ago is unlikely to have currency value today.

One thing that all versions of a CV can have in common is their structure. One structure is offered here, but this is by no means the only one. Some readers may be surprised that it appears, at first glance, to be the wrong way round. Most people, on the front page of the CV, include all personal details, name, address, etc. Pause for a moment to think about this. In the situation of a job application, the purpose of the CV is to get you an interview (the interview then gets you the job!). When the person who is shortlisting for the post is looking through the CV, what is being sought is a vignette of the applicant, and that individual's ability, not details of home address etc. Capitalise on this; use the first page for impact and include:

Managing self – making it work for you

On page 1

- Name, qualifications, and current post.
- Any roles/experiences that are unique to you outside your current post (e.g. advisor to another organisation, chair of a professional group).
- Key personal skills, strengths and attributes which describe you, and which are worded to match the organisational culture in which the new job is based (e.g. effective communicator; understands the importance of working within resource; effective change agent; can work within a team, etc.). Present these in a bullet pointed list to give it impact and to catch the eye of the reader.
- Two or three sentences that capture what you have to offer to the profession/organisation. For example, 'I can bring to the organisation in-depth knowledge of 'x', enthusiasm and ability to get the job done through motivating my staff'.

On page 2

- Current post .... (wef 1st June 1997)

Responsibilities and achievements include:
Try to write these as outcome statements, rather than just *describing* a part of your role. For example: (a) initiated and coordinate a journal club within the unit. As a result the unit has a collection of review notes on relevant topics which act as a resource; or (b) led an outreach service to support renal patients in the community. As a result, the number of readmissions to the unit has decreased by 20% over a period of 6 months.
　　　Finish with ....
　　　My current post gives me .... (one or two sentences)

- Previous post .... 1st July 1995–31st May 1997

Responsibilities and achievements
You can include a little less detail here, and the detail will get less as you move backwards in time.
　　　Finish with ....
　　　The focus of this post was ....

- Previous post .... 1st August 1991–30th June 1995

Responsibilities and achievements
Finish with a sentence highlighting the key issue of this experience.
　　　If your career goes back more than 10–15 years, in most circumstances it is only necessary to refer to your earliest experience in brief terms, for example January 1970–March 1976: various posts at staff nurse grade.

Enhancing and developing your career

● Career breaks

There has been a lot of debate about this issue – should career breaks (usually in relation to women) be recorded in their CV? The feminist view may believe that there is no need to explain/apologise for a break. A more pragmatic view is to include a statement something like: 'during the period January 1990 to May 1995 I took a career break'. This ensures that the potential employer can track your experience, and this is important in ensuring safety for patients and clients. Many organisations and managers positively welcome those people with some life experience, as this brings an added dimension and balance to the workplace.

On the final page
Your final page should include the 'nuts and bolts' about you. A layout is suggested below:

● Personal details

Name	*Date of birth*
Address (home)	*Tel/fax; mobile/email*
Business address (if you want to include this)	*Tel/fax; email*

● Educational and professional qualifications (listed in reverse order)
● Professional body membership (e.g. Member – Royal College of Nursing)
● Publications
● Current studies
● Personal interests and activities include .... (two or three sentences is usually sufficient)
● You may also like to include your referees here, with their contact details, having first alerted them to your intentions.

The first rule of CV writing is to have 'one you prepared earlier'. Often, when you decide to apply for a job, the turnaround date for applications is quite tight. You need that time to do your information gathering about the particular organisation, so having a CV ready to adjust, rather than having to start from scratch, is a real bonus.

Prepare your CV on good quality white or cream paper, and use a basic, plain typeface and black ink. Resist the temptation to use graphics and colour. Unless you are in the world of the arts/media, this is considered inappropriate and it can cause problems in reproducing your CV. Many organisations now scan CVs to copy them; coloured ink and elaborate graphics do not survive this process well.

PROACTIVE PERSONAL DEVELOPMENT PLANNING – A KEY TO YOUR FUTURE

The value of preparing and maintaining a PDP has never been more apparent than today. In the health care industry, as in others, the picture of career profile, career portfolio and career development has changed dramatically – and it is a more complex process than many believe.

Every bit of your work and life experience can contribute to your future career. Activities undertaken during career breaks, or during time when you are working abroad or not working in health care, can offer something of value to your future. The structure of the 'portfolio' career has been formalised, and is now valued for its eclecticism, rather than being labelled fragmented and piecemeal.

However, the important thing is for *you* to take charge of your career – don't assume someone else will do it for you. For example, if you see an opportunity at work, once you have done your homework about what it entails, and how it might fit into the 'big picture', put yourself forward, make a suggestion about how you might tackle it. In this way, your own personal development is contributing to the wellbeing of the organisation, and vice versa. This is how it should be. Development is about doing things 'on the job', as well as about studying formally. PDPs should be congruent with the organisational development plan – in that way the optimum outcome derives from the effort everyone puts into a project (see also Application 4.2).

The timeframe for your PDP is important. Five years is now considered long term; normally the medium term is considered to be 3 years, and 1 year is a short-term view. This has arisen because of the rapid and continuous pace of change in the world of work. It is too easy to be shell-shocked by this, and think that planning is futile because by the time one has developed a plan, it is irrelevant because the world has changed. This gives the clue to how to prepare your PDP. Keep it flexible and responsive. The portfolio of experience that nurses and other health care professionals are required to produce in order to remain in practice is an excellent basis for your PDP. Preparing this gives you the opportunity to

Enhancing and developing your career

reflect on what you have done, what you enjoyed and what you think you are good at. Remember to capture your experience as well as your courses.

When looking ahead, try not to think in defined roles. For example, it is not helpful to think that in 3–5 years' time 'I want to be a xx'. The way things are changing, it is unlikely that there will be a post called xx, and in any case, different organisations call the same post different things. Be open to opportunities that present themselves. One danger of planning too far ahead is that you overlook exciting things in the here and now.

The thing to do is to make a note of the sort of things you would like to be doing in your role in 1, 3 and 5 years' time. For example, you may say you want to work in a team, or in an autonomous post; you may prefer to be in a big hospital or in a remote community. When you have collected this information, you may find it helpful to skim the job advertisements in a number of professional journals. Do not look at the job title – look at the *description* of the job and match it to your 'wish list'. You may get a surprise, and begin to look at different roles in different contexts.

Another important activity when working on your PDP is to consider, objectively, your strengths and development needs. Brainstorm these on paper. You can then consider ways on how you can capitalise on your strengths, and ways in which you can develop those skills and knowledge areas you have identified as priority. Be careful not to fall into the trap of thinking that you must do a formal course for everything. Some areas of development are best achieved by shadowing a colleague. For example, if you think you are weak on chairing meetings, ask a colleague whom you feel is good at chairing if you can sit in. Then watch the *process* of meeting management (normally we concentrate on the *content* of the meeting). Make notes on what you felt worked well and why, and try it out for yourself.

A mentor can be a good resource to help you to consider different career opportunities (see Chapter Six). This is not the same sort of relationship you may have had with your allotted mentor/preceptor on the ward. Clearly it is important that you feel comfortable with your mentor, so you should take time choosing the right person. Your mentor does not have to be from the same professional background as yourself – in fact sometimes someone outwith your professional group can provide a fresh perspective. You may only need to visit this person two or three times a year, so you may choose someone from another area of the country. You may meet your mentor as a result of networking.

STRUCTURED NETWORKING

Structured networking is an excellent and cost effective way of developing your career and tapping into a plethora of resources relevant to your area of practice. Most people find that they are networking automatically, but you may find it helpful to consider one or two basic activities as a way to develop your networking skills further. Always keep a note of telephone numbers and addresses of people you meet. This may be from conference attendance, people who have visited your place of work, or people with a high professional profile you feel could contribute to your development. Providing you have a focused objective, you will find that the majority of professionals are happy to give time to others, and in fact many more senior/experienced people see this as an overt responsibility. Should you wish to contact someone whom you do not know personally, either write to them, or telephone their personal assistant, explaining who you are and how you feel the person can help you. You must be very focused and succinct. Ask for a 30-minute appointment. Be on time, take with you your questions, and wind up the interview within the allotted time. Be sure to follow up the meeting with a 'thank you' letter.

Keep contact details of those who have published an interesting article in a journal. If you feel you would like to ask a question, write to them. Professional groups, such as the Royal College of Nursing specialist fora, offer a good way of networking with people who have similar professional interests. However, remember that people from different backgrounds can bring very different and refreshing perspectives.

The key points to remember are: be proactive, be focused, be reliable and be prepared to give your time to others when approached.

Acknowledgement

This chapter is reproduced from Churchill Livingstone's Dictionary of Nursing, 18th edition, 2002 (ISBN 0 443 06483 0), Appendix 8 (p. 512–518), by permission of Elsevier Ltd.

Enhancing and developing your career

Discussion questions

- Look at your current CV. Does it tell the reader what you want them to know about you, your skills, strengths and attributes? Is the content focused and relevant to the focus and recipient of the CV?
- If you do not have a CV, note key points that you wish to emphasise when preparing a CV. You may find it helpful to show it to a trusted friend or colleague – and ask – do you recognise me here?
- How can your CV enhance your chances of securing an interview?

Reference

Department of Health 2003 Agenda for change, the new NHS pay system – an overview. Department of Health, London

Chapter **Ten**

The interview:

securing the position

Jo Ouston

- Factors you can and cannot control
- Preparing for interview
- Question and answer dialogue
- Weaknesses and strengths
- Attending for interview
- Listening skills

OVERVIEW

Now Ouston takes you through the next stage of applying for that job – the interview. She offers some tips for preparation and how to deal with the interview on the day.

INTRODUCTION

You have submitted such a good curriculum vitae (see Chapter Nine) that you have been selected for interview. Whether you are being interviewed for a promotion or a regrading or a new position there is a number of common factors that apply:

- The interviewer(s) want you to be good/to match their needs.
- It is your responsibility to demonstrate this.
- You need to know that the job/promotion will suit *your* needs.
- There is nothing you can do about any rivals you may have.

There are also factors over which you have no immediate control such as:

- the style of the interview
- the length of the interview
- the questions you will be asked.

It is all too easy to spend time in advance of the interview worrying about things you cannot control instead of preparing yourself to give of your best in the areas you can control.

So here are some tips about how to prepare yourself for the interview.

PREPARING FOR THE INTERVIEW

Application form/CV/letter of application/ assessment forms

The interviewer(s) will have one or more of these in front of them on the day. They should have read what you have submitted/know to be there and if so will doubtless have questions to ask about it. You should make sure that you know this material inside out. If you do this, no question based on it will throw you, other than perhaps the banality of some of them, so be prepared!

The person and job specifications

The key task of the interviewer(s) is to establish whether you match the role/position in question. Your task is to help them. You do this by giving them facts, by telling them of relevant achievements and experience.

You should do this not only when invited but also in response to probing questions. It is quite reasonable for interviewers to probe, but important for you to understand that they don't want to catch you out – they would much prefer to be reassured that they have nothing to worry about in the area they are probing. Remember that only facts reassure.

Questions: specific and general

You know or can work out many of the questions specific to the role that you will be asked and you need to prepare answers that are *brief, positive* and *reassuring.* You must also have questions of your own, which should relate to areas where you might hope to be challenged or stretched, or where you might have particular opportunities to use your key strengths.

Questions and answers create dialogue, but in an interview the result can be a very stilted and one-sided form of dialogue. You can help to avoid this in two ways. First, think of 'dealing with questions' rather than simply answering them. Second, try to follow up your answers with related questions that you want to ask.

There are a number of general questions that come up frequently at interviews. Three favourites are:

- Tell me/us a bit about yourself (notwithstanding your CV/application form!).
- What is your greatest weakness?
- What is your greatest strength?

The subtext behind these may be anything. Be aware that sometimes interviewers ask questions without quite knowing their own purpose. However, you should answer the first with a straightforward sales pitch and the second with a demonstration of self-awareness, which will reassure the interviewer that there is no weakness that will affect your ability to do a first-class job. Your strength should be genuine too, and relevant to the job. Do not feel you are 'blowing your own trumpet'. It is important that professionals are self-aware, and can present a balanced view of their ability.

The sales pitch should last about 90 seconds and should include:

- a brief résumé of your career (they already have all the details, remember)
- one (maximum two) brief career highlight(s) or achievement(s)
- what you bring to the role (i.e. key abilities/skills/experience)
- what kind of person you are, your attitudes/principles (if not included above).

Remember, no false modesty. They want you to be good!

Any weakness must be genuine (this way a strength is often implied) and it must not be relevant to the job, thus:

- 'I can get over-fussy about (am good on) detail.'
- 'I am not good at admin.' (There is no administration in the job.)

Preparing the above and doing thorough research on the department/organisation/people will repay handsome dividends and increase your level of confidence enormously before the interview.

The interview: securing the position

Remember not to talk too quickly – this is something we do when we are under pressure, so, be aware of how quickly you may be speaking.

AT THE INTERVIEW

Having prepared as thoroughly as possible, you are ready to discuss the post/move/role. You should imagine it as a *discussion* or *dialogue* between you and others to determine whether there is a match, whether you and the role fit each other. There is another fit to be aware of. How would you get on with the new people with whom you might be working? Ultimately the judgement of the interviewer(s) about this will decide whether an offer is made. It is not a question of discriminating in favour of someone who is liked over someone who is competent. Almost invariably when several people are interviewed for one position several of these *could* do the job. There will, however, be a natural gravitation towards anyone who seems to match or complement the team already established.

Listening

This is the key, and it means much more than hearing spoken words. Imagine that you and the interviewer(s) are enveloped in a huge, transparent, plastic balloon. Your aim is to be conscious of what is going on. Not self-conscious, which tends to lead to paralysis, but aware. You don't need to be aware of anything outside the balloon. Listening starts with paying attention – to tone and body language as well as to the words. You should also listen to how you are being heard by the interviewer(s). Do the responses mesh with what you are trying to convey?

As you become more aware of what is going on you will be less self-conscious, so that when you do not understand a question you are able to say: 'I'm sorry. Do you mean X or Y?' or even 'I didn't understand that question. Can you repeat it please?'. This is so much better than starting to answer the wrong question.

In any case you are not supposed to know everything. Indeed one of the questions most frequently asked by interviewers relates to concerns that the job might be too easy for you. You might get bored and leave within a few months, or do a poor job because the job provides no stimulus. If this or any other negative point is true, do your best to reassure the interviewer(s). Get offered the job and turn it down later.

CONCLUSION

Always be aware that to some extent, you are interviewing the interviewer(s), who, in this context, represent the organisation. It may be that your experiences at interview lead you to believe you would not be happy doing the job. It is just as important to know what you do not want to do, as what you do want to do!

Discussion questions

- How can you prepare effectively and efficiently for an interview?
- What can you do to ensure you make a positive impact at interview?

The interview: securing the position

Index

Note: Page numbers in *Italics* refer to tables, those in **bold** refer to figures and boxed material

Index

Index

Index